Noseworthy

Barbara Caplan-Bennett

Noseworthy

This is a work of nonfiction.

To contact author Barbara Caplan-Bennett:
Website: https://www.facebook.com/Noseworthyamemoir
Email: noseworthy2020@gmail.com
Twitter: www.twitter.com/Noseworthy2020

To contact Hilltop30 Publishing Group, LLC:
Website: www.hilltop30.com
Email: tombrew@hilltop30.com
Twitter: www.twitter.com/tombrewsports
Phone: (727) 412-4008

For multiple copies of this book or to arrange book signings and/or speaking engagements, please feel free to email or call Tom Brew at Hilltop30 Publishing Group, LLC.

Printed in the United States of America.

<u>DEDICATION</u>

For My Aitchy,
Paul Caplan-Bennett

You are my best friend, man of
my dreams, love of my life.

You are my soft place to land and
my strong rock on which to lean.

I would never have survived this
journey intact without you by my side.

I love you so very much.

— Barbara Caplan-Bennett

Once Upon A Time

My nose has always been my Achilles heel.

When I was 12 or 13, it grew a little too big.

When I was 14 and horsing around with friends, I got dropped on my face on a cement floor. I'll never know if the noticeable bump on my nose was the result of genetics or of that fall – or both.

When I was 15, the cutest boy in our class was sitting behind me in the school auditorium and when I turned to try to catch a glimpse of him, he said in a loud voice, "Hey you, turn around, I can't see. Your nose in the way!" He laughed, then his buddies all laughed. I was mortified.

When I was 16, my mother offered to pay for a nose job, because everyone was doing it. "You'd be so beautiful if you just got your nose done," was her plea to me. I heard: "you're not beautiful the way you are." Not exactly the message you want from your mother. It left an emotional scar that I bore for years. And because I was obstinate and did not have any intention of giving my mother the satisfaction of being right, I decided I was fine the way I was. I would never get my nose done!

But I wasn't fine the way I was. And never is never really never.

So, in my late thirties, when a friend went to work for a plastic surgeon, I found myself open to the possibilities. There were enough medical reasons for insurance to cover it and the reduced cost was hard to pass up. At 39, I decided it was time to stop being stubborn and admit my mother had been right. I wanted a new nose, and I got one. My mother was so happy and she didn't even have to pay for it!

But as is typical when one chases perfection, I wasn't content with my new nose. It wasn't quite symmetrical. My nostrils didn't seem quite even, and the bridge seemed a little too high. Of course, those were the things I always saw when I looked in the mirror. Still, it was a vast improvement over the nose I was born with.

One night, at the ripe old age of 40, I was stopped at a red light on a warm summer night. A guy in the car next to me tooted his horn, and when I rolled down the passenger window, he yelled "You are so beautiful!" That was all I needed to hear. My nose wasn't perfect, but it was good enough and I was happy.

My life moved forward. At 41, after years of failed relationships, bad dates and long stretches of being single, I finally met my match. Paul and I clicked immediately and because we were both in our 40's, we didn't need to do the long dating dance. We knew what we wanted, and we wanted each other. We married the following year and lived happily ever after.

That should be the end of the story, but of course it's not.

*** *** ***

Within a few years, I needed surgery on my nose again. I had developed congestion in my sinuses that was affecting my ears, and medication wasn't clearing it up. The ENT doc wanted to remove some polyps and trim the turbinates in my nasal cavity to remedy the situation.

Not a big deal, and when I recovered, I could breathe better than I ever had in my entire life. OK, nose, are we all good? Are you done screwing with me now?

*** *** ***

But no, my nose was not done. When I was my early 50's, a fleshy bump appeared on my nose. It would get irritated then heal, then get irritated again. I didn't like the look of it. I didn't like the feel of it. I wanted it gone.

"It's nothing," the dermatologist said. "A little scar tissue."

The law firm where I worked had just changed insurance carriers and this was a doctor I had never seen before. What he was saying didn't add up. Why would I have scar tissue suddenly out of the blue. "Who knows?" was his answer. He gave me cortisone cream that would "clear it up" and sent me on my way.

But it didn't clear up and my instincts told me something was definitely wrong. I went back to my primary care doc and asked for a referral to a different dermatologist. "I read the report," my doctor said. "It's nothing."

"But it gets irritated, then heals, then gets irritated again. Isn't that what cancer does? I'm telling you this thing is weird and I want another doctor." I was not taking no for an answer. Being a good guy and a good doctor, he listened to me and acquiesced.

That one moment of assertiveness, that one moment of being my own advocate may have saved my life.

*** *** ***

I sat in the office of my new dermatologist. She walked in, took one look at me and said, "let's biopsy that." I felt relieved that I wasn't crazy. What I should have felt was worried.

The biopsy came back with an odd diagnosis. It showed

two cancers – both squamous and basal cell carcinoma. The doctor admitted it was odd to have two different cancers in one place, but not unheard of. It would be fine, she assured me. I would have the Mohs procedure and all would be well.

For the uninitiated, the Mohs procedure is one whereby they cut the smallest piece of skin possible to remove the tumor, then view it under the microscope to see if they got clean margins. If they did, great. You're done. They sew you up, maybe do some minor plastic surgery to minimize the damage, and that's it. If there's one edge of the margin that is not "clean," they go back in and take just a wee bit more, but just in that one spot. Then they check again. Now clean margins? Great, you're done. Not yet? Back for another slice. It's a rather ingenious way to keep from having to simply cut a giant chunk out of someone's face to ensure having gotten all the cancer.

I had the Mohs and all went well. It took two rounds to get clean margins, then they pulled a flap of skin on my nose to cover the hole where they'd removed the tumor and voila' – I would be good as new.

***   ***   ***

Except that I wasn't. The nose I had bought and paid for would never be the same. I now had a dew-drop shaped scar that created a divot in my nose. Everyone said, "no one will notice except you." But I did notice and I was back to being self-conscious all over again. It took a good year for the scar to heal and eventually I adjusted, as one does. Truth be told, even with the odd little dent, it was still better than my original nose.

Over time, though, it became obvious that the divot wasn't going to be the only issue. Despite using sunscreen religiously, the skin on my nose started to discolor. While all this had been going on over the previous five years, I had given up my long–time job as a Legal Assistant and had reinvented myself as a space designer working for a closet company designing closets, garages, home offices, etc. The change in my work life, once again, meant a change of insurance and doctors.

While my previous diagnoses and treatment had been done by doctors at Cedars Sinai in Beverly Hills, I was now covered by Kaiser Permanente. The dermatologist I saw at Kaiser seemed fine. She assured me the freckling on my nose was from the scar tissue of the Mohs. It was "nothing to worry about." But I should be sure to wear sunblock – which I already did. Unlike the first wrong diagnosis years earlier, I believed this one. I shouldn't have.

*** *** ***

As time passed, the discoloration grew larger. It was weird but not horrible. It still just looked like freckling or that I had tanned unevenly.

One evening while attending a wedding, someone said to me, "You have chocolate on your nose." What? How could I have chocolate on my nose? I went into the bathroom to check and realized they were referring to a small dark spot on my nose where the scar tissue was. I dismissed it. Just freckling. Nothing to worry about.

Over the next few months, it became a constant refrain from people around me – you've got something on your nose – you've got dirt on your nose – you've got ink on your nose – you've got chocolate on your nose! (Everyone knew I loved chocolate. They must have thought I was shoving my face into a bag of it and inhaling my fix.)

At this point, I was due for my yearly visit with my dermatologist. I was going to return to the doctor I'd already met, but Paul had recently been seen by Kaiser's Head of Dermatology for his yearly skin check-up and raved about what a great doctor he was. Unfortunately, Dr. Goldstein was in high demand and I couldn't get an appointment with him for several months. What did a few more months matter? I wasn't worried about anything this time; I was just annoyed by the stupid freckling and was hoping to get it removed.

*** *** ***

By the time I walked into Dr. Goldstein's office, it had been a full nine months since the first "chocolate on your nose" comment at the wedding, and fourteen months since my last dermatologic full body check.

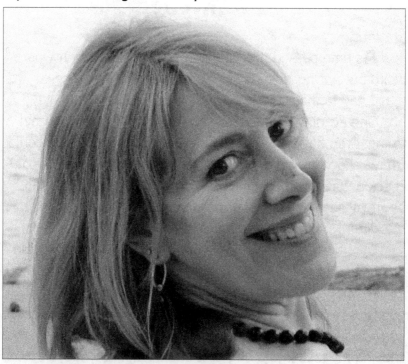

Chocolate on My Nose? Nope, Melanoma!

Dr. Goldstein lived up to Paul's hype. He had a stellar bedside manner – kind and thorough, with a sense of humor. He asked why I had come in. I gave him a brief history and he checked the notes in the computer. Then I said, "this dark spot is so annoying. I don't care if I have to pay for it myself because it's cosmetic. I want you to make it go away!"

He put on his little magnifying specs, turned on the bright light, took a good long look at it and said, "I'm afraid we need to biopsy that."

I shouldn't have been, but I was shocked. The other doctor said it was just freckling. But that, of course, was before the dark spot had become so prominent so as to provoke such frequent commentary. Still, why hadn't she warned me of the potential danger? How many wrong diagnoses was I going to rack up? I was on my fourth dermatologist, the Mohs specialist and his pathologist. And here I was again, back at square one.

Dr. Goldstein sent me to their best plastic surgeon for the biopsy so my scar would be minimal. But once again, the nose I bought and paid for was going under the knife.

The pathologist confirmed it was not freckling. It was melanoma. Melanoma! Mela-fucking-noma! A kind of pretty word for a very ugly cancer. Back then, melanoma was considered deadly. It was one of the top five cancers for low survival rates.

But I was lucky. The pathologist said it was "only" melanoma in situ – basically Stage 0, noninvasive. All good things, important words that translate into "no big deal." And there was a simple procedure to fix it. They would send me to their Mohs specialist.

Ah, Mohs, my old friend! A familiar word. Not fun, but manageable. I would spend a day with the Mohs guy, then I would return to the plastic surgeon, and all would be well.

***   ***   ***

But all wasn't well.

My consult with the Mohs specialist was daunting and depressing. Turns out, melanoma is not a one-day Mohs like other skin cancers. They can't simply look at it under a microscope to see if clean margins had been achieved, as they had with basal and squamous cell skin cancer. If I understood it correctly – and I'm not sure I did – they have to freeze the tissue they remove so they can stain it to see the melanoma cells. In other words, this was a long, drawn-out process. One day at the doctor's, then off a day while they freeze and stain. If they didn't get it all, you go back again the next day, then another day off while they freeze and stain.

My Mohs specialist did not sugarcoat anything. He was brutally honest and told me the area he would have to remove would be extensive and that he was uncertain if plastic surgery could return me to my original state or even close to it.

Basically, he was going to take most of the skin off the top of my nose and they might have to take a flap of skin from my forehead to cover the damage. He said the color match of the skin flap might not be good and he couldn't or wouldn't say how bad the end result might be.

My now dear nose, the nose I bought and paid for, the nose my husband fell in love with, the nose I wanted to grow old with, was going to be scarred – really badly scarred. The little dewdrop divot I had so fretted over seemed cute in comparison. And I wouldn't know just how bad it might be until it was all over.

To further complicate things, once the Mohs process began, the area on my nose would remain an open wound, because they don't close and fix it until they know all the cancer is gone. And although the wound is bandaged, activity is severely restricted to prevent bleeding. I could not do anything that would make my blood pump harder. I couldn't work. I couldn't play. Once we got started, I couldn't do anything but sit around and wait.

Paul and I were scheduled to leave the following week for a long-planned vacation to Yosemite. My doctors agreed waiting a couple of weeks would be fine so we could have one last hurrah. We left for vacation with heavy hearts, but vowed to enjoy ourselves before we would have to return to face the music.

*** *** ***

It was a terrific vacation – a gift from the universe. Everything swung our way for that one week. Yosemite's waterfalls were at their most beautiful, thanks to a winter of heavy snow. The weather was perfect. The crowds were manageable. Areas of the park that were still closed from the heavy snowfall magically opened just as we arrived so we could see them in their greatest pristine glory. It was the most incredible run of good luck we've ever had on a vacation.

I have seen many of our country's national parks in my life. Yosemite, at its best, is by far and away one of the most majestic and spiritually powerful – the perfect antidote for our fears and anxieties. Paul and I were filled with gratitude for the good fortune that came our way when we needed it most.

Still, as great as it was, I admit, as I washed up before bed each night, I spent a fair amount of time staring in the mirror at my nose, uncertain as to just how bad it would look when all was said and done. I thought I was facing a worst-case scenario, that this was as bad as it could get.

I was wrong.

*** *** ***

I began the Mohs procedure the Monday following our return from Yosemite.

On Tuesday, I received a call. "We didn't get it all. Come back tomorrow."

On Wednesday, the doctor took another slice of my nose. I wondered how much more they could take. The skin that ran almost the entire length of my nose was already gone.

On Thursday, the phone rang. I answered with fingers crossed that he got it all, but I somehow knew he didn't. What I didn't know, what I couldn't have guessed, was what he said next. The pathologist's findings showed the tumor ran deeper than they thought, deeper than the Mohs procedure could handle. He was referring me to Kaiser's Head and Neck Surgeon.

I didn't understand. What did that mean? My imagination could not even run wild enough because I had absolutely no clue what the next step might be. I knew only one thing: I was desperate to get in to see this surgeon guy as soon as possible. I wanted answers. I needed answers.

Looking back, I'm surprised my usually overactive imagination didn't come up with an idea of what was to come. But it didn't. This was just a tumor on my nose. It just couldn't be that big of a deal.

But you know what I'm going to say next.

I was wrong.

*** *** ***

I had to use all my powers of persuasion to get the appointment scheduled quickly. And when I finally walked into Dr. McNicoll's office, I was instantly overcome with dread. I don't know why it hadn't hit me so hard until that moment, but stepping into that waiting room was truly terrifying. I still didn't know what to expect, but my instinct told me it was going to be bad. I grew nauseated as we sat there and waited.

And waited. And waited.

We waited for over 45 minutes, and I grew more anxious and sick to my stomach with each passing minute. We both grew antsy and angry at the long wait, but there was nothing we could do.

I should stop to mention, at this point, that Paul was my constant companion throughout this process. He attended every appointment with me, found ways to distract me, amuse me, make me laugh. He reassured me that I was beautiful, no matter what.

But as he and I sat together in that waiting room, even he could not distract me. He didn't even try. It wasn't until much later that I thought about what that wait must have been like for him. Suffice it to say, neither of us could have imagined the journey upon which we were about to embark.

*** *** ***

Dr. McNicoll was a tall, gentle soul with a quiet demeanor. Somehow, he managed to be forthright and honest, but comforting at the same time, a gift not many surgeons are blessed with. He finally put a name on what I had – Desmoplastic Melanoma – a difficult to diagnose form of skin cancer because it doesn't always present as the typical black mole. It can be amelanotic (no color) and is commonly mistaken for scar tissue.

Yup. The original dermatologist who said it was just "scar tissue" had likely missed it all those years ago, and although I'll never know for sure, I would put money on the fact that I had probably had melanoma from the start. When something is labeled "difficult to diagnose," it stands to reason it took that many years and at least eight different doctors and pathologists before someone finally figured it out. But thank goodness they did!

The hallmark of desmoplastic melanoma is that it is slow to metastasize (the good news) but is locally extremely aggressive (the bad news), which is why it came back even after my original Mohs years earlier.

Dr. McNicoll calmly laid out my options:

I could let him surgically remove a chunk of my nose and maybe he'd get it all, but maybe not. The upshot was that there was a high probability it would return, and they would have to take more. And every time they took another piece of my nose, it meant another surgery, another patching-up and still, it could return. And in five years, Paul and I might be discussing how to spend my "remaining time," because eventually it would metastasize, and once it did, my chance of survival was slim to none.

Or, I could let him remove my whole nose. My WHOLE nose. All of it. Gone. Completely.

There's even a name for it. A full rhinectomy. And if I let him amputate my whole nose, the chances were excellent that they would completely get it, once and for all. One and done. They would set me up with UCLA to create a prosthesis that would glue on or clip on, and I would go on with my life.

He looked me in the eye and said, "it's your decision."

Then he looked at Paul and said, "If you want to be enjoying lunch with your wife in ten years, your best shot is to let me take the whole nose."

I cannot describe the level of disbelief Paul and I both felt upon hearing this.

This is not like being told they have to take a piece of my lung or my breast, or schedule chemo or radiation. Those things are truly horrible, of course. But we all know others who have gone through that. We have a point of reference.

But to cut off my entire nose? Who ever heard of such a thing? What would that even mean? Would I just have a giant hole in my face? Would there be a skin flap over it? I just could not wrap my head around it. To say I was completely and utterly numb is an understatement.

Dr. McNicoll told us to think about it, discuss it at home, and call his office with our decision so we could schedule surgery.

*** *** ***

We left his office in silence. We rode the elevator down to the street in silence. We walked out outside and crossed the street to the parking structure in silence.

I stopped walking finally, turned to Paul, and in the middle of Sunset Boulevard, completely broke down. We stood, holding each other, crying together, unaware of passers-by or traffic, or the world around us in any way.

You'd think I was scared because I had cancer. Not just any cancer, but a deadly cancer. But all I could think of was that I was going to be a freak.

A freak without a nose.

*** *** ***

Paul and I had a big decision to make, but we pretty much knew what was going to happen. We spoke with another melanoma specialist and others, and the consensus was all the same: with melanoma, to cut is to cure.

The decision seemed to be made by my diagnosis. And once I made the decision, I just wanted the whole damn thing over with.

A surgery date was scheduled – July 5, 2011. The following days were spent in a flurry of pre-op appointments and tests – scans, blood, x–rays. Every day for two weeks, I kept my shit together. I met with doctors and technicians and I wore my brave face.

And every night around 11 p.m., when Paul and I crawled into bed and turned on the TV, I would break down in sobs. Paul would turn off the TV, hold me while I cried, talk to me about my fears and feelings and sometimes cry with me.

Every. Single. Night.

*** *** ***

In one of those discussions, an interesting question arose that changed my spiritual belief system forever. I always believed in karma, and still do in many ways. Paul and I had studied Kabbalah a few years prior, which teaches that everything that happens to us is the result of something we did in this life or in a past life. Kabbalah, as we were taught it, embraces a belief in reincarnation. Basically, the karma always comes back eventually, even from a different existence.

As I sat in bed and cried, I said to Paul, "I keep asking

myself what I could possibly have done to create this?"

My wise and wonderful husband – who had embraced the Kabbalistic teachings far more deeply than I had – looked at me and said, "Nothing. You didn't do anything to cause this. Sometimes shit just happens."

I looked at him, a little shocked to hear he felt that way, and felt a great wave of relief. I am not a perfect person. I've made plenty of mistakes in my life. I've hurt people, I've been mean and selfish at times. I've been self–absorbed and arrogant. But I could not imagine I had ever done anything that would warrant permanent disfigurement as a punishment.

As for past lives, maybe they're real. Maybe they're not. I don't believe we are even meant to know the answers to such questions. I just know that we are here in this life now. This life is our responsibility. This life is all we have to work with and it's up to us to make the most of it. If reincarnation is real and I did something shitty in a past life, well, I can't change that, can I?

So, no more blaming the victim. I had not caused this, except perhaps by spending too much time in the sun. It wasn't the karma coming back. Shit had just happened.

And I would come to understand through this experience that shit happens to everyone. Bad shit. Horrible shit. No one is immune. That person that seems to have the perfect life? They don't. Or maybe they do right now, but with rare exception, they won't always. Very few people, perhaps none, get to the end of their lives without having to endure some kind of hardship, some kind of trauma.

I had the good fortune to get through 57 years of life without anything beyond the typical emotional pain we all go through – losing parents, break-ups of relationships, job losses, etc.

Until this. Was losing my nose going to be my Waterloo? Or was I going to be a phoenix and rise from the ashes?

I didn't yet know. I just had to get through the days ahead and worry about the future later.

*** *** ***

As the day of surgery approached, I had the daunting task of telling all the people I knew and loved, as well as my employer.

My bosses were amazing. My managers, Jose and John and even our vice president, Mary, were understanding and supportive and just wanted me to get well and return to work when I was ready. It was a huge relief to know I wasn't going to be jobless on top of everything else. Of course, since I had a job that involved sales and direct client contact with strangers every day, I had no idea how I was actually going to perform my job without a nose, but I would cross that bridge when I had to.

Telling my family and friends was harder. It was a shocking thing to say to someone, "they have to cut off my nose." That much I knew. What I didn't anticipate was that I would be putting myself in the position of comforting people. I didn't think about the fact that people would be frightened and worried that they might lose me. I didn't expect people to cry, but cry they did.

It was up to me to tell everyone I was going to be OK, even though I had no idea if I was going to be OK or not. But I understood. I wasn't upset with anyone for being emotional, for being scared. I knew it was because they loved me. In some weird, twisted way, it was comforting.

Several friends were cancer survivors who had lost breasts to cancer, and they were the easiest people to tell.

They knew the journey in front of me and had the best things to say.

One of them warned me that I would lose friends over this. I thought long and hard about who in my life might possibly disappear because I had cancer, and I couldn't think of a one who wasn't steadfastly behind me. But she was right. I did lose someone – a family member. There are always those people who are too frightened by illness or death to step up. The excuse is always the same. "I'm afraid I'll say the wrong thing." So, they offer up an email saying, "thinking of you." But then they don't check in, they don't follow up, you never hear from them again. They just simply disappear.

This I don't understand. Perhaps I am too hard on people, but this is where I am unforgiving. I've known people who faced tragedy of all kinds – they've lost body parts, they've lost husbands at a young age, and worst of all, I've known someone who lost a child in a most unthinkable way. When it happens to someone you care about, you don't get to worry about saying the wrong thing. You just show up. If you care, if you love someone, you just fucking show up.

But I had been warned, and it was only one person. It made me sad for a while. But I've accepted it and moved on. And the flip side is that every other person in my life showed up big time.

***   ***   ***

Besides Paul, I have the great fortune to have my big sister, DeeDee, and Vicky, my best childhood friend of over 50 years. Both were solidly in my corner, two women standing ready to do anything and everything I needed that would be helpful, backed up by a bevy of close friends and family.

If ever there is a testament to the value of loved ones, it's when you're about to get your nose cut off to survive cancer. And they all want to know how you are and how you are managing every step of the way.

And that's where the Caring Bridge begins.

I don't even remember now who suggested it. I think it was my niece, Sara. Caring Bridge is a website where people who are going through a medical crisis can post updates for everyone to see. It means that the person or their family isn't constantly having to contact everyone individually to let them know the most recent developments. There's just one post that everyone can read at their convenience.

This seemed like a brilliant idea to me. But I had so much on my plate, so many things to take care of pre-op, that I didn't want to have to figure out how to start it, so I called upon Sara, the closest thing I have to a daughter and little sister, all rolled into one. She was happy to create it for me, because people who love you want to help. They want to have things to do, tasks that will make them feel better, like they are contributing to your recovery.

And voilá! I had a Caring Bridge page.

What follows are my entries as I lived through the next ten months. There are a few early entries written by Dee-Dee, as noted, so neither Paul nor I would have to deal with it on the day of surgery and just after. Her posts and some of mine are simple updates, perfunctory information. But as I recovered from surgery, the emotional experience took center stage, and I was so grateful to have a place to put my thoughts and feelings, and even more so to read the comments and encouragement of others who followed my story. It made a life-altering experience something positive and meaningful for me as I went through it.

I share it with you now.

Caring Bridge Entries

July 1, 2011, 9 p.m.

Dear Friends and Family,

Most of you now know, I have a rare form of cancer called desmoplastic melanoma, also called a "spindle tumor. The good news is that the cancer has not spread. If we conquer it now, I stand a good chance of being around a long time. The bad news is that spindle tumors are very aggressive locally and require radical treatment.

On July 5, I will have a rhinectomy – which means they will completely remove my nose. This is my best chance to have a full recovery. "To cut is to cure," as the saying goes. (Hmmm, a little poem, sort of.)

The prosthodontist – yup, that's a word – is creating a temporary plastic nose for me to wear after surgery. I'll cover it with a bandage and hopefully it will tide me over until I get an actual prosthesis from UCLA sometime this fall. Reconstructive surgery is no longer looking like a viable option. A prosthetic nose is not a perfect solution, but they look incredibly real, and most people won't even know.

Lucky for me, I am blessed with the most incredible husband on the planet, close-knit family, understanding and compassionate bosses and a boatload of supportive and loving friends – that's you.

This is all quite overwhelming and neither Paul nor I may be able to return all your emails and phone calls in a timely manner. So, I've asked my niece, Sara, to create this page where you can check in when you wish to see my progress. My sister, DeeDee, will keep it updated until we feel up to tackling that ourselves.

It's going to get weird, folks, having a big hole in my face. I'm as vain as the next guy, so I'm not quite sure what my mental state will be after the surgery, but I know a lot of people are rooting for me, and that makes all the difference. Thanks for all of your love and support. And watch this space.

A Note Before My Surgery

July 2, 2011, 10:40 a.m.

After a week of never-ending doctor appointments and pre-op tests, I'm looking forward to spending the weekend getting the house in order and relaxing. My nose's last night will be spent watching fireworks at Dodger Stadium.

I have such mixed feelings about all of this – dreading it, and at the same time just wanting to be on the other side of it all. By year's end, I hope to be back to leading a normal – albeit altered – life.

I want you all to know that the surgery itself is not complicated – a walk in the park for my surgeon, who has done many rhinectomies over his 30-year career. If I'm really lucky – and if the anesthesiologist is good – I'll be alert enough to get out of bed and use the bathroom within a few hours, in which case they'll let me come home that very day. My nose – the cavity, that is – will be packed and bandaged. A temporary clear plastic nose form will be bandaged over that. Ironically, it's a similar process to when I had my nose done nearly 20 years ago.

I should not be in a lot of pain – just not very comfortable because of the packing.

They will be grafting a thin piece of skin from my thigh to the edges of where my nose was, so that the space heals properly to allow a good fitting for my prosthesis. I'm told the skin graft is actually more painful that the rhinectomy. Remember what it felt like when you skinned your knee as a kid? It's like that.

OMG, seriously? Listen to me rattling off procedural details like this is so ho-hum. Suddenly I'm struck by the absurdity of it all. As my friend, Kathrin, says, I've entered "cancer world." Sadly, I know many of you out there are all too familiar, having dealt with it yourself, or watched a loved one's journey.

I hope this is not TMI. But many of you have questions, and to me, knowledge and information are power. The more one knows, the easier it is to deal with. It's the unknown and uncertainty that are truly frightening.

Just know that I will be going into that OR on Tuesday feeling very cared for and supported by all of you. The sheer power of love coming my way is palpable and will certainly ease my path.

XOXO, B.

P.S. – Those of you that know me as Bunny from my childhood are free to use it. I know I will always be Bunny to many of you. If you didn't meet me until adulthood, however, don't even try it.

Here's What Helps

July 3, 2011, 10:34 p.m.

Reality is starting to bear down pretty hard as Tuesday approaches. Daytime is manageable, nighttime, not so much.

Here's what helps:

The Cats – Nothing like a purring ball of fur nestled against you. (A purveyor of smiles in the daytime too. William just stole the plastic hospital band I accidentally left on the counter after tests the other day. A new toy! Yippee!)

Valium – Way better than Tylenol PM. Oh my God, Valium, where have you been all my life?

NPR – As fascinating as it is by day, that's how medicating it is at night. They run the BBC at midnight. Nothing brings on sleep faster than a bunch of droll Brits droning on about what's happening in parts of the world I've never heard of, especially combined with the Valium.

Paul – Always and forever, but now even more so. His tolerance level of my needs right now is staggeringly high. Whatever I want, whatever I need, the answer is an unhesitating "yes."

If Tuesday didn't loom so large, I could get used to this. But, alas, it does.

A Complete Breakdown
Can Be a Good Thing

July 4, 2011, 2:52 p.m.

For those of you who think I'm some kind of super-woman, well, today the real breakdown finally came. I've cried plenty, but until today, had not just let it go – cried, sobbed completely and unabashedly – until it was all done. And even when I thought it was done, there were more tears still.

I must admit, it felt like a huge release. To cry long and loud, to say to Paul over and over how much I don't want this to happen to me was like dropping a heavy load.

The completely fucked-up part is that even after I drop the load, it climbs right back on me again.

So now I'm back to just wanting it to be over. The suspense is horrible.

I've been unsure whether going to Dodger Stadium tonight is a good or bad idea, but I think if I take plenty of Kleenex, I'll be alright. I'll sit with my Aitchy, the love of my life, on a beautiful summer evening, facing the mountains, and somehow, I may find a little peace before the morning comes.

How apropos – Todd Rundgren's "Just One Victory" just came on my iPod. It's been my battle hymn in troubled times before. Once again, it'll be my rallying song. Now I have to go cry some more. But this is a song that makes me raise my head up and stick out my chin in defiance, even while the tears flow.

See you all on the other side of tomorrow.

Fireworks Light Up My Spirit

July 5, 2011, 12:04 a.m.

So glad I went tonight. Had I stayed home, I would have probably spent the night crying. Instead, I laughed and spent time with my Aitch and two dear friends, Bubby and Schmavey – Michael and David to the rest of the world. Things almost felt normal. The Dodgers lost, but that's about as normal as normal gets these days.

And then, there was gorgeous, spectacular, stupendous, magnificent fire in the sky!!! As I sat watching, I resolved that next year, I will be in those seats again relishing the fireworks, as I have every year for 24 years running, and all of this will be well behind me.

Love to you all. Goodnight.

Surgery News

July 5, 2011, 1:55 p.m.
By DeeDee Widdes

Bun (Barbara) is out of surgery and in recovery. She'll be there about an hour and then Paul will be able to see her.

The doctor said they found no negative surprises when looking at the tissue initially, which is great. Pathology reports after the fact will tell the full story.

Looking for CLEAN MARGINS. He felt that the surgery went well. I will get more information from Paul after he's seen her. Hopefully home to her own bed by tonight. Let Great Healing begin!!

The Amazing Bunny (Barbara)

July 5, 2011, 7:58 p.m.
By DeeDee Widdes

She's home! While I was talking to Paul, she said she wanted to talk to me – is she amazing or what. She's still a bit groggy and not real comfortable but managing and so happy to be home and have this part behind her. She said that her spirits are actually pretty good. She's relieved at this point and will deal with the emotional side of it later. As Scarlett O'Hara would say "I'll think about that tomorrow."

Below is medical information Paul got from the doctor following her surgery:

"They did not find any surprises in the tissue. They did take some of her nasal bone but smoothed that out. This is so it is in the best shape possible for the prosthesis to sit comfortably. They did a skin graft from her thigh that the doctor said went very well and was smaller than he originally thought. The thigh will heal in time but is sometimes the cause of more pain than the nose. We will see him next week to have her bandages changed. And yes, he did use the plastic mold of her nose so it looks like something is there under the bandages, as opposed to a flat look."

Speaking of the new look, she says she looks like someone put a big old knife in the middle of her face, and she could now have a part in a Freddy Kruger movie. Her sense of humor is still intact. She does want all to know what really wonderful care she had today and how much that helped her get through today's experience.

Hoping you have a good night tonight in the loving care of Paul. Signing off for tonight. One of us will do an entry at some point tomorrow.

Post-Op

July 6, 2011, 1:27 p.m.

Well, it's me again! Yesterday wasn't actually bad.
The people at Kaiser were absolutely amazing. The anesthesiologist did a great job – didn't OD me and included some
anti-nausea stuff in my drip. The last thing I remember
before surgery was someone asking if I'd ever had morphine
before. I felt a wave of euphoria and I was out.

I was thrilled to come home. I'm not really dealing yet
with the emotional side because I'm so bandaged, I have no
idea what's going on under there. The wound is weeping,
which is annoying as hell, but normal. Today, I don't feel as
good as yesterday. My throat hurts from being intubated,
I have a headache, my stomach is rumbly, and my leg is
tender where they took the graft. The one thing that doesn't
hurt is my nose – or where my nose was. Though in the
middle of the night I did have a phantom itch on what
seemed like it should have been my nostril.

This is probably not my most creative piece of writing.
I don't feel terribly clever at the moment. But I know you'll
all understand.

I look like shit. Can you say shit on the Caring Bridge
site? My eyes are swollen, piggy eyes, my hair looks like
some weird flat rat's nest, and I'm carrying five pounds
of water from the IV. Yes, I got on the scale, just for fun.
That's dissipating, though.

This morning, it was Bailey the Cat who gifted me with
a hairball (I guess they are taking turns), because what
Paul really needed right now was someone else to clean
up after.

And speaking of my darling Aitch. He is – no surprise – waiting on me hand and foot and keeping me under tight watch so I don't overdo. To quote what's-her-face from On Golden Pond (oh yeah, Katharine Hepburn): He is my knight in shining armor. I forget the rest of the speech. Chalk it up to drugs.

And special thanks to my sister, DeeDee, for all her help, too. I'm very lucky to have a big sister. She taught me how to read before I ever went to school. She played with me, babysat me, protected me. OK, she also beat me up, destroyed my Raggedy Ann doll (long story), and took a piece of my ear once when cutting my hair – but nobody's perfect.

I always extoll the virtues of my wonderful husband, but she deserves big kudos as well. So, thanks, Big Sis – I love you.

And thanks to all of you for your wonderful notes on my guestbook. It really lifts my spirits. And though right now I'm under the influence, I know reality is going to hit home very soon and reading over these messages will buoy me when I need it most.

I won't know about clean margins for another week or ten days, but keep the energy coming – CLEAN MARGINS!

XOXO to all

Short But Not Sweet

July 7, 2011, 2 p.m.

Struggling today. Feel like crap. Might be the fact that Monday night's Dodger dog is still rumbling around somewhere in my system. (TMI?) I was warned the anesthesia might do that.

Had a rough night. But my hero ran out for me at 7:30 a.m. to get some stuff from CVS that I'm hoping will "move things along." Poor guy. He hasn't had a good night's sleep in days.

Sorry I don't have something cheerier or more profound to write. But my head hurts too much.

The Journey Ahead

July 8, 2011, 3:31 p.m.

Yikes! A very tough 36 hours, but now it is behind me and happily so. My entire digestive system went to the gates of hell and back again. All I can say is that the guy that gave birth to the monster in the movie "Alien" ain't got nothin' on me.

I've turned the corner now and starting to feel better. Tomorrow night is our monthly poker game at our house, and I'm desperately hoping to be able to sit up at the table long enough to get in some hands of poker with my guys. I look completely hideous and terrifying, but I'll be in safe company with guys who know me and love me, so I'll be OK.

I'm still able to hide behind my bandages.

But now that the worst of the physical part is behind, I'm starting to grapple with the emotional loss. I'm still having trouble fully grasping that when everything comes off my face next Wednesday, there will truly be nothing there. I can actually see a couple of edges of where the hole is beneath the dressing and it completely freaks me out.

It seems absolutely unimaginable not to have an actual nose. I know so many people who have been through various other cancers and accidents and have lost body parts. Hey, I live with a three-legged cat! But I don't know anyone who is facially disfigured. And to think, everyone makes a big deal out of Tina Fey's tiny scar.

OK, so I was never a Madison Avenue beauty, but I always felt attractive or cute enough to "present well." I've always taken care of myself to stay that way (witness the multitude of moisturizers and eye creams in my bathroom).

So how will this change me? I know that it will. How can it not? I just have to find a way – some way – to be sure I grow from this and not shrink from it; for the former will surely help me keep the best of "me," and the latter will mean the loss of who I truly am.

Yet shrinking seems the easiest thing to do. Close the door, turn out the lights, hide away.

And it may be fine to indulge that urge somewhat while I'm adjusting. But I absolutely, positively must not stay there.

I will need everyone's help to do this. I don't even yet know what that means, or how anyone can help, because this is so much in my own head. I know that my Aitch will love me no matter what. I don't doubt that for a minute. But I do feel bad for him that the face he fell in love with will no longer be there. Regardless of his assurances, that's got to be hard for him.

The cats are really the only ones who will not "see" me any differently. Not for one second. As far as they're concerned, once I'm back to my usual duties of feeding and litter box–cleaning, not a thing will have changed for them.

I guess I will just have to dig really deep and try to find that place in me that always likes to say: "It'll be an adventure!" before I embark on something new. (Well, if you don't know me, I do often say that when faced with the unknown.) I'll try to find my way to that place. But I'm not there yet.

For now, I'm just going to focus on the fact that I'm physically feeling better. The rest will come soon enough.

Thank you all for your wonderful comments. You have no idea how much they mean to me right now.

All Over the Map Today

July 9, 2011, 5:52 p.m.

Can't stand being in bed another minute, but don't have the strength or energy to do much.

Going forward with the poker game tonight, crazy as that seems. I need something for my sanity, which is in a great state of flux today. Have no idea whether it's a good idea or not – I may last one hand or a bunch of hands, but I have to give it a go!

As for my head space: The whole "dreading getting the bandages off" is over, and I've passed over into "I can't wait to get these things off my face." It's kind of like how I felt about surgery. In my imagination it's going to be so unbelievably horrible to see myself for the first time that I just want to be past it so I can start to deal with it and move on.

I remember feeling this way both times when my parents died. I just wanted to jump over the hard part and be on the other side of grieving. But I've been through the grieving process enough times to know that the only way to the other side is directly through the fire. And the fire won't come until Wednesday when the bandages come off.

Anticipation is a wicked, wicked form of torture.

But here's the little tidbit that made my day. Paul let me feed the cats for the first time this afternoon. The sheer normalcy of that act was enough to make me weep. Normal seems so utterly out of reach at the moment. God bless the cats for giving me that. Wish me aces. That will help.

A Tribute to My Motley Crew of Poker Buddies

July 10, 2011, 5:52 p.m.

Today is a good day, because last night was a great night. If there was any question about whether playing poker was the right thing to do, that question has been answered – in spades! (Unfortunately, not the ace of spades.) I did not have great poker hands last night, but I did have a great time.

We've all been told about the healing power of laughter, but if any further evidence was needed to support the theory, last night's game was excellent proof.

First, I am so very grateful for my guys. You know you're in for a fun night when you're playing with guys named Schmavey, Bubby, Dr. Chewy, my Aitch, Eug and Steve. OK, we clearly need to find a nickname for Steve.

They were, each and every one, absolutely pitch perfect in what I needed last night. They were kind and gentle about my appearance, but showed me no mercy at the card table. We laughed long and hard about all the ridiculous usual crap we laugh about every month at these games. The night was not about my nose, but there was no avoidance of it either.

When I got a little pale around the edges, they made me lay down and rest, but while I was at the table, I was expected to be on my toes or suffer the usual barbs hurled at any slacker who spaced out during betting.

In short, I lost $12, but I would gladly have paid it many times over for a Night of Normal. I loved every minute of it. Heartfelt thanks to my Guys. I love you all dearly.

L'Chaim!

July 11, 2011, 10:54 p.m.

Short entry tonight. Very tired. Got up and about a bit today. Hard to believe how quickly I get exhausted.

But I do have one tale to tell. Today I received a beautiful gift from my husband – a literal gift, not just the abundance of figurative gifts he gives me daily.

A few days before my surgery, we stopped in a local shop on 3rd Street and I saw a very delicate, rather artistic Chai necklace. I've never worn a Chai, but somehow felt very connected to this one. We left the store and I thought about it repeatedly, until I finally mentioned it to Paul, who had been on the other side of the store when I saw it.

Today, he gifted me that Chai necklace, which now hangs around my neck close to my heart.

For those of you who are not familiar with the symbol, "Chai" is the Hebrew word for life, as in the drinking toast, "l'chaim" – "to life." Chai is also the Hebrew symbol for the number 18, believed to be of great spiritual importance and good fortune in Judaic numerology.

When I learned this as a child, it gave me a little buzz of pride, because my birthday is on the 18th of June, and also because my Hebrew name is B'racha, the Hebrew word for "blessing." So, I was born on the day that's the symbol of Life and good fortune, and I was given the name of Blessing. And indeed, I've always felt I've been living a very Blessed Life.

This necklace means so much to me because going through this ordeal, it would be quite easy to lose sight of that fact. I asked Paul to please, please, help me remember, no matter what happens in the months to come, no matter how hard it gets, I am still leading a Blessed Life.

This beautiful gift will help me do that. Thank you, my dear Aitch.

P.S. For Esther (and everyone else who has asked or wonders about why I call Paul "Aitch"), here's the Cliff Notes version to answer your question: Years ago, I was home with a cold and saw "Sleepless In Seattle" on cable for the millionth time. The little girl in the movie uses initials for everything instead of names. So, in a silly moment later that day, I called Paul "Aitch" (H) instead of "Honey."

The rest is history.

T-minus 24 and counting

July 12, 2011, 7:07 p.m.

A weird day. Anticipation creeping in. Tomorrow looming. No more mystery behind the bandages. It will all become stark reality.

Just a warning to everyone. Please no calls. I plan on going into full "radio silence" mode while I grapple with whatever bizarre array of feelings descend upon me.

I have some doctor appointments in the a.m., but the bandages are not actually coming off until the afternoon.

This is the hardest part. Not just for me, but also for all of you, my friends and loved ones. Because I know this is where you will all want to help but will not really be able to. This, Paul and I must face alone – just the two of us.

I do know you are all out there, and it means more to me than I can tell you. Some of you I haven't seen in years, some of you I don't even really know, you know me only through Paul, some of you are friends since childhood, and some of you are newer arrivals to my life. But I appreciate knowing each and every one of you are all out there with your good wishes and prayers. That's all you can do – but believe me, that is so very much.

Until I re-emerge, love to you all.

Fully exposed

July 13, 2011, 5:51 p.m.
ByDeeDee Widdes

Just got a text from Paul. They are home from the doctor after seeing what the aftermath of the surgery looks like. To quote Paul "we laughed and cried – we are mostly OK."

This doesn't change Bunny's declared "radio silence" until she's ready to reach out. I'm sure they have an emotional roller-coast ahead of them.

They have a long journey and as her big sister, I'd like to add my thanks to all of you who have been so supportive. I know what it means to both of them.

DeeDee

The Good, The Bad, and Definitely The Ugly

July 14, 2011, 11:36 a.m.

This is going to be a long one, and pretty much "just the facts, ma'am." Not ready to delve into the emotional side, but I know people are wondering about some things, so here goes:

The Good

1.) The best news is that the deep tissue margins are clean, meaning I don't have to have any more of my face removed. This is a huge relief, as you can imagine.

2.) My smile is back! For the past week, whenever I smiled, my upper lip didn't move to expose my teeth and I wasn't sure if it was because of the bandages limiting movement, or because something about the rhinectomy had actually altered how I smile. Completely freaked me out, so I'm thrilled to say that my smile looks normal again.

3.) So far, the skin graft appears to be healthy and healing well. This is huge, because a failed skin graft really sets back the entire process by months.

4.) I can finally breathe with my mouth closed, so I can sleep without waking up every half hour to moisten my parched palate.

5.) I have come to adore my doctor, a man of great compassion and expertise – an unusual combination in a doc. He is also sending me to a Kaiser melanoma specialist out in Riverside just as another source of information and to check into any further steps to keep the melanoma at bay.

43

6.) Yesterday afternoon, after the shock passed, I experienced a kind of euphoria, probably relief that the most horrifying part was over, and I was suddenly seized with the urge to plan – trips, crochet projects, social events. Yes, that did pass (see below).

7.) Something has happened that I never thought possible: Coming through this ordeal with Paul has actually deepened our love and strengthened our bond in a way I couldn't imagine. There are no words even close to sufficient to describe the admiration, respect, gratitude and love I have for this amazing man in my life. That's all I can say, because mere verbiage is inadequate.

The Bad

1.) The surface margins were not clear, i.e., on the very uppermost layers of epidermis, there are still cells showing melanoma in situ (the earliest stages). Fortunately, the upper area near my eyes is all clear. They are only showing up in the horseshoe around where the bottom of my nose was. My oncologist and pathologist are conferring to determine whether or not an additional surgery is necessary just to take that very top layer of skin and graft another piece. I hope this is not necessary, because it will slow down getting my prosthesis. But I've come this far, and I'll do whatever I've got to do to make it all go away.

2.) I still don't know whether I'll need radiation. My oncologist told us that some oncologists have an "always" or "never" policy with regard to melanoma. But Kaiser has what he called a "50/50 approach," meaning they review each case individually and determine the best course of action.

3.) More waiting, more wondering.

The Ugly

At the risk of eliciting a barrage of "you're beautiful" comments on my guestbook – none necessary, thanks – at this moment in time, the "Ugly" is me. Don't contradict me on this one, folks. I'm looking in the mirror and it is a serious freak show. That said, Paul and I are oddly OK with it around the house.

Last night, as often happens when we get into bed and the distractions are gone, I was beset finally by my grief. There is no more "Cute Bunny" or "Come Hither Barbara," there is a new me, one I have not yet adjusted to.

Physically, I can't even describe how bizarre it is not to have a nose. I'm having a lot of phantom sensations, and several times I've actually raised my hand with the intent of scratching my nose or picking at something crusty feeling inside my nostril – yes, we all do it – but there is NO nostril!

Paul and I have been chronicling this in photographs and I've been debating the question of posting. But I don't think I'm ready for that yet. And for the more squeamish among you, it would certainly have a high gag factor.

I am comforting myself with the fact that this is the worst it is going to look. The whole thing is angry and in-flamed with stitches and dried blood, crust and other kinds of gunk. The doctor said that eventually the whole crevasse will settle down and become like the rest of my skin, except where the actual hole itself is.

So there's the story for now. As I said, no great emotional delving for the moment. Not ready to go there with all of you yet. But a clinical description, I thought, would be a good way to start.

And I guess, if I want to find a bright side, there are more things listed under the "Good" than the "Bad," and that counts for something!

Long Day's Journey
Into Pinkberry

July 15, 2011, 9:08 p.m.

Long day, short entry, but I always say that, don't I?

Took a shower – a tricky endeavor involving saran wrap strategically taped to my face. But oh, how delicious it was to stand in a stream of hot water, even though I couldn't put my head fully under it. The littlest things are sometimes the most sublime.

Got restless, but didn't have the get-up-and-go to do anything.

Finally, when Paul came home, I put on my temporary fake clear plastic nose and let him drive me a block or two from Pinkberry so I could have a short walk for a treat. Went to the Farmer's Market sticker store next door and bought some stars and butterflies with which to decorate my temporary fake nose just for fun.

Exhausted now, going to bed. A decent day. Still, I wish I could wake up tomorrow and discover it was all a nasty dream. I may sound all fine and dandy, but I'd give almost anything (except Paul) to have my nose back. Ain't never gonna happen. Yup, the witching hour tonight is going to bring a good cry for sure.

Where Has All the Clever Gone?

July 16, 2011, 10:15 p.m.

No wit, no wisdom, no nothin' tonight.

Had my first "girl date" this afternoon with my dear friend, Nancy. A simple walk for a few blocks (a little longer and farther than yesterday) and little bite of lunch together. Sounds easy peasy, yeah? After she left, I laid down for a "little rest." Two hours of sleeping like the dead later, I woke up feeling like I'd spent ten hours digging ditches. Poor Paul was back to serving me dinner in bed.

Man, I just don't recognize my body right now, absence of nose notwithstanding! I seem perfectly fine, until I try to actually do anything. You'd think I'd had major surgery or something!

But it was wonderful to have a visitor, someone I trust who has walked her own cancer path. Thanks, Nance. A good, safe place to start for re–emerging into a social life.

Sweet dreams, all.

*** *** ***

P.S. I wore a tiny flower and a tiny ladybug sticker on the bandage over my TFN ("temporary fake nose"), and when I asked Paul his opinion, he said, "Well, it kind of calls attention to it." Then we both got a good belly laugh out of that one – as if without the tiny stickers, no one would ever notice the giant weird bandages in the middle of my face.

Good one, Aitch!

Lessons Learned
and 'Bad Teacher'

July 17, 2011, 8:02 p.m.

Lots of learning going on today. First, I think I may have cracked the code on how to properly put on the TFN – Temporary Fake Nose for all future references. I have to cut the surgical tape in a very specific shape and actually use two different size bandages over that.

There are still a few bugs to work out. One of the band-aids started to come off about two hours in so I think I need a better quality band-aid, and after wearing it for three hours, I did start to accumulate condensation inside the plastic nose. Lord, that sounds so weird.

The other lesson is what wears me out and what doesn't. Turns out, being up and about isn't really the worst culprit – it's actually relating to people that's exhausting. I don't mean that in a bad way. It's just more tiring to interact than not. Today we went to see a movie, and sitting in a theatre for two hours did not tire me out the way talking with a girlfriend did for an hour or two. But of course, that makes sense. Relating to another human requires an exchange of energy that watching a movie does not.

We saw "Bad Teacher" because it was easy and stupid funny, and because I have a personal affection for Cameron Diaz (warning: name-dropping about to occur), since I used to know her through my old job and she was always so sweet. Brilliant movie-making? Not even close. Good light fare for someone not entirely up to full intellectual speed yet? Yes, indeed.

Finally, the best thing that happened (actually yesterday when I was out with Nancy): A little boy on the street looked at me, and after a little beat, smiled a beaming smile at me. Not a mocking smile or an embarrassed smile, but a genuine friendly smile. I wondered what made this boy different than a little boy that I completely freaked out a few days ago. I must have looked terribly frightening to the little guy.

Actually, I don't think it was the two boys, but rather other things that were different.

First, I was wearing the stickers when I saw the second little boy, and I actually think that was what made him smile – because the silly lady had stickers on her nose! The other difference, possibly, was me, and how readily I smiled at the second little boy; whereas I was still nervous when I crossed paths with the first.

I'm slowly learning to be around people with this thing on my face and not be conscious every second that it's there. It's not very comfortable, but it is manageable. Right

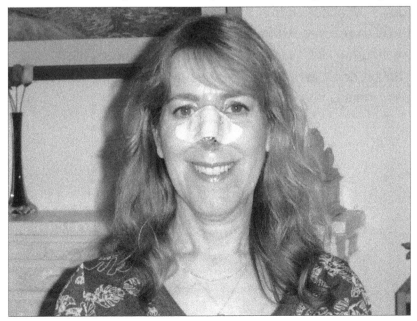

The Infamous "TFN"

now, it's the only way I can manage not being a hermit.

Finally – after a pretty normal day today – tomorrow I re-enter "Cancer World" for my appointment with the melanoma specialist. I'm bracing myself to hear more difficult news, but hoping I will be pleasantly surprised.

By the way, for those of you who have mentioned some form of mental health support, no urging necessary. Rest assured, I'm still having visits with the oncology therapist. My occasional rounds of therapy over the past 30 years changed my life dramatically for the better, and two of my closest friends are therapists. It's an excellent tool and one I've never shied away from using. So, please, all know that I am taking care of my mental health as well as my physical health.

OK, I think I just hit my wall. I'm done for the day. Tomorrow, it's back on the merry go-round.

P.S. – Paul and I actually had a minor disagreement today! Woohoo! Normal life! It was absolutely delightful. I was so relieved we finally had five minutes of him treating me like "Normal Wife" and not "Cancer Wife." Though don't get me wrong, the pampering that "Cancer Wife" gets is very addictive.

More Answers, More Questions, and Flying Monkeys

July 18, 2011, 10:03 p.m.

Had a terrific meeting today with Kaiser's top melanoma guy. He was wonderful, spent over an hour with us, explained things in great detail, even had a sense of humor.

Here's what we know: My cancer is Stage II (that's good). My chance of survival at five years is about 80 percent – though he was very emphatic about the numbers not meaning much, but rather every person is an individual and stats are meaningful only up to a point. Still 80 percent is also pretty good.

My chances of having a new melanoma are just slightly higher than anybody else. My chances of recurrence are hard to define, but he gave us – yes, both of us – a rigorous lesson in checking my body and advised we do it monthly.

He recommends doing an additional surgery to try to get all of the remaining melanoma in situ cells. Remember that "in situ" means it's not actually cancer yet. They are the precursor to cancer, but to leave them there is just asking for a recurrence. As he put it, I've come this far, why would I not want every cell gone." That said, another surgery is my best chance of getting it all, but not a guarantee. He said radiation is a very last resort. He felt that the risks to it were many (affects your smell and taste and makes you a lousy candidate for further surgery because you are basically burning all the tissue to kill the cells). But in the interest of full disclosure, he said it's possible that surgery still won't give us clean margins, and then we are definitely looking at radiation.

So, it seems like a pretty settled deal that I will have another surgery and not radiation with the slimmest, tiniest chance that radiation may still be necessary down the road, small enough so that I felt optimistic.

I arrived home feeling pretty good about it all, then got a call from my surgeon's office to let me know they had scheduled me to be seen by the "tumor board," a group of doctors – radiologist, chemotherapist, hematologist and oncologist – to discuss my further treatment.

This referral was actually ordered last week, before my meeting with the melanoma guy. I'm seeing my surgeon on Wednesday and will discuss with him then if being seen by the tumor board is still necessary.

The whole idea of a "tumor board" freaks the shit out of me, frankly. I loved my doc today, and I love my surgeon. But I have great trepidation about being passed around from doc to doc to determine what they're going to do to me next even though they don't know me. I'm well aware that this is a completely irrational and emotional response, and that I'm probably lucky to be seen by the board and have still more experts considering my fate. But it just feels absolutely overwhelming.

It's like I'm standing here at the beginning of the yellow brick road. I've already come all the way from Kansas on a twister, and my prosthesis is down there in the Emerald City, and the frickin' witch keeps throwing obstacles in my path. The TUMOR BOARD feels like the flying monkeys are coming to get me and carry me off to a dark land far away from the beautiful synthetic nose that is my ticket back to normal life.

It's been a very long day, and since I am exhausted, I'm also a bit emotionally raw. It's a long road. I know that. I have to keep putting one foot in front of the other. I will eventually get there. My patience is just a bit thin today is all. Tomorrow will be better.

The highlight of the day was stopping by my office at Closets By Design, which we were literally passing right by on the way home from Kaiser. It was wonderful to see the smiling faces of my bosses, John and Jose. It reminded me what I'm trying to get back to. It's a good thing when you love your bosses. Not everyone has that, and I'm very grateful, indeed.

Every day has good things in it. Sadly, it's human nature for the bad things to get all the attention, but I'm working like a dog to try to find the light in each day.

An Abundance of Gifts

July 19, 2011, 9:40 p.m.

Today was certainly a better day, for so many reasons. Perspective, a good night's sleep except for the 5 a.m. hairball – Bailey's, not mine. What is it with him waking us at 5 a.m.?

But it was mostly a better day because of my gratitude for the abundance of gifts I've received these past few weeks. I've steered clear of this topic until now, because I don't want anyone to feel obligated or weird or embarrassed or uncomfortable in any way. But the truth is, since the day of my surgery, I have been inundated with gifts.

Some people sent books, gift cards, CDs of various comedians, a beautiful shorty robe, fruits and nuts (yummy), homemade soup and banana bread (also yummy), and flowers (gorgeous, but with today's delivery we've used up every inch of available space out of the cats' reach!).

A little birdie told me a care package of my favorite skincare products is on the way (just in time as I'm running out of everything and not ready to face the department store).

And one especially enterprising friend delivered a great meal and a pedicurist. This last gift was especially appreciated because everyone who has touched me for the past two months has poked me with needles, prodded me, cut me. It was sheer heaven to have someone massage my feet and legs and make my toes all pretty!

But these are the tangible gifts. Just as important have been the many beautiful entries in the guestbook that have moved me to tears, given me back my sense of worth, offered great words of wisdom or hearty laughs (sometimes all those things in one note!).

And one of my favorite gifts (not that I'm picking favor-ites), was a large card with the face of a kitten on it – very adorable, of course – but the thing that made it a favorite was because my friend had taken a little band-aid and placed it over the kitten's nose. It was addressed to "boo-boo kitty." Simple, yet moving and funny all at the same time.

But even if you have never made a guestbook entry, never sent a card or a single thing my way, if you are read-ing this, you are giving me a wonderful gift, indeed. Not all of you know that I'm a "recovering writer," meaning I'm a life-long writer who hasn't been writing much these past few years. For me to be read, well, that's just about the best gift you can give a writer.

Granted, getting cancer is the cheater's way to accumu-late readers. But writing these journals each night has done me so much good on so many levels. Most of you don't know that I have literally 22 notebooks filled with journaling from my teen years all the way into my 30's. I don't know why I stopped. I only know how good it feels to do it again.

So, thank you – all of you – for the abundance of gifts, both corporeal and intangible. Each and every package, card, guestbook note, prayers or "juju" you've offered up on my behalf and your sheer presence out in cyberspace reading these posts, are all immensely appreciated and so valued. They have all helped speed my healing and ease the way on this bumpy road. You are all amazing people of compassion and empathy, and I'm filled with gratitude to have you in my life.

Two Steps Forward, One Step Back ... or Sideways?

July 20, 2011, 8:08 p.m.

Saw my surgeon today. The skin graft is healing up quickly and nicely, which was great to hear. But discussions and information made me even more confused, if that's possible. And I got so much info today, I can't possibly spit it all back in this journal.

But here's what I loved about my doc. He said the reason I'm confused is because it is confusing. The doctors are confused. Melanoma is very unpredictable, and it's not like there's a "right" answer. Everyone takes their best shot at guessing the best thing to do. He urged me to go ahead with seeing the tumor board, which I will on August 5.

He's doing a bit more research with two other doctors about the question of surgery and whether or not it would be a big deal or a small deal. If it's a small deal, I will definitely move forward with it. If it's a big deal, we will revisit the subject after the tumor board despite what the melanoma expert said.

So here I am not having a clue as to my next step, and unable to get to my end goal of getting my prosthetic nose, without knowing the path there. And I just have to sit with it and be OK, a most difficult challenge.

But all things considered, I'm doing OK. I'm actually dipping my toe back into the water with closet clients next week. Small stuff, simple stuff with clients I already know. Stuff that doesn't take great energy or stamina, which is still in short supply, but slowly returning.

As for the hole in my face, it's actually shrinking, which is normal and expected as the swelling goes down. The doctor cleaned it up a bit and I'm getting quite adjusted to seeing myself in the mirror now.

I can feel life slowly returning to normal daily patterns, and that's comforting. Not sure if I'll have much to say on a daily basis for a while, as the barrage of changes and events is slowing down. But then, I always seem to have something to say – whether or not it's worth saying is another story! A trait that appears to be hereditary – a blessing and a curse.

In the meantime, it's Wednesday! I'm going to lose my troubles in the two-hour episode of "So You Think You Can Dance!" Better than drugs.

Until next time.

It Don't Come Easy

July 21, 2011, 10:10 p.m.

Last night I made a decision. I have several weeks before I know what I'm facing next. As you've all witnessed, I do not do well with waiting these things out. Since this is a rather lengthy "holding pattern," I decided I am just going to live each day as if there were no further decisions to make. I'm healing, feeling better, getting a little stronger each day.

There are lots of things to do. My desk is a disaster area, my work papers need organizing, I have clients to see next week, and of course, there's daily napping that must be attended to. I have plenty to occupy me and that's what I'm going to focus on for now. Easier said than done, but that's the plan.

So today was going just swell. I actually sat at the dining room table, iPod in ears, and worked on designs for a client, which felt wonderful! I did a couple of follow-up calls, and had a short walk and lunch with a friend. I was ready to pass out into oblivion, when I made the mistake of opening the mail.

Apparently, the State of California has the weird idea that I'm currently getting paid my full salary even though I haven't worked in weeks (I'm not), and therefore, they have determined I do not qualify for disability checks. Say what? I was told last week that everything was completely in order and my checks (they now owe me five) should be arriving shortly.

During the best of times, this would annoy me, but these are not the best of times, and my reserves for deal-ing with stupid bureaucratic bullshit seem to be just about empty. Of course, it was too late in the day to do anything about it, so now I have to sit with it until tomorrow. Like I need one more thing to worry about.

Paul, of course, reassures me and says everything will be fine. On an intellectual level, I know that it will be. This is actually a little, silly thing that should be easily rectified. I wish my cancer could be so easily dealt with. But when everything already feels hard enough, I just gotta wonder, WTF?

All I know is that tomorrow, I will muster up as much energy as I can to turn into what my family lovingly calls "Herschel Caplan's Daughter" (cue dramatic music!).

If you knew my dad, no explanation is necessary. He was a force to be reckoned with, and he taught his daughters to be the same way (a true women's rights advocate before it was popular).

Know what you want and ask for it. Start gently, start nicely, but get tough and pushy if nice doesn't work. If you get an idiot on the phone, ask for the supervisor, and whatever you do, don't back down. But most important, when all else fails, use the Herschel Caplan "Voice of Authority," the tone that says, "don't f*ck with me because I will take you down!"

That knowledge has served me well over the years.

So, look out State Disability Office. Tomorrow, Herschel Caplan's Daughter will be giving you a call ... and you better be ready!

Now, if only I could handle my cancer that way. Hmmm, maybe I can. Maybe I am?

Bureaucratic BS, Part II

July 22, 2011, 10:30 p.m.

Exhausted tonight but didn't want to leave everyone with a cliffhanger regarding my disability.

Apparently, if there is any tiny little problem, rather than calling or sending out a letter that says there is a tiny little problem, the state just sends you out a notice saying you don't qualify. Hmmm, isn't that like putting out a candle with a fire hose?

I called my very nice representative, who is so nice that she never bothered to call me back. I'll give her the benefit of the doubt. Maybe she was out today. It is, after all, a midsummer Friday.

So, I called the main 800 number. Only was on hold for ten minutes and got a nice gentleman who informed me they were just missing some forms – the forms I faxed ten days ago. So, I refaxed to a new number and per the guy's instructions, marked my paperwork "HARDSHIP." Seriously? Is anyone filing for disability not suffering a hardship?

Here was today's bright spot. I got a call from my office. My amazing bosses saw yesterday's journal entry about the disability blip and got in touch with the company's HR person, who called me just to ask how she could help! Between my husband, my doctors and my bosses, I could not ask for better care!

Adrianna and I worked through some things, and I discovered she'd never received any paperwork on me from the state. No paperwork, no checks, so it was back on the phone to the state. This time on hold for over half an hour. Turns out, they sent the paperwork to the wrong address.

However, to their credit, both guys I spoke with were very kind and reassuring that they would do their best to get this all figured out so I could start getting my checks ASAP.

I want to believe in magic, I really do, but Tinkerbell is fading and at this point, no amount of hand-clapping is going to bring her back. Only that lovely check in the mail can do that now.

So "Herschel Caplan's Daughter" barely got a work-out today, but I suspect she will be called forth again in the not-too-distant future.

Yawn. Bureaucratic BS is boring. But I'm too tired to write a new entry now. As Herschel Caplan would say: "Schlaf Gesunderheit," everyone – Yiddish for "sleep in good health."

Credit Where It's Due

July 23, 2011, 2:35 p.m.

I had lunch with a wise friend yesterday. She asked if it was hard for me to be told over and over that I'm brave, inspirational, amazing, etc. She wondered if it wasn't an awfully hard image to live up to.

The answer is that yes, sometimes it is. To me, I'm just me, warts and all. Like any good batter, I'm just swinging at whatever pitch life throws my way, trying to "stay alive" at the plate. And I strike out plenty.

Cancer hasn't made me Superwoman. It has simply forced me to face certain harsh realities. I know there are those people who would crawl in a hole if this were happening to them, but I'd put my money that most of you out there would step up if you were in my position.

But here's the real crux of the matter. I can say with great certainty that there is one thing and one thing only that has been the source of my strength, that has given me the ability to put a smile on my face, to joke about the most horrible things, to have the desire and will to get up every day and face whatever I have to face. There is one thing without which I would want to throw in the towel, hide away or crawl into a hole and not come out.

That one thing – or I should say that one person – is my amazing husband, Paul. My dear Aitch. The love of my life. The man of my dreams. I don't mean to paint him as a saint, though in many ways he is. He is not perfect, but he is perfect for me.

He has never, for one minute, allowed me to feel alone or unsupported. He has held me and bolstered me, wiped my tears and talked me "down from the ledge" when my fears start to get the better of me. Most importantly, he has kept me laughing. He has an innate sense of when to let me be sad and acknowledge that I have every right and reason to be sad or angry about how my body has betrayed me, but he also knows exactly when to drop the one–liner that will bring me around to a smile again.

If he were not by my side through this, if he were not my partner in life, I'm telling you without a doubt, that I would not be the brave, amazing, inspiring, (blah blah blah) person that you all seem to think I am.

I would be a terrified, depressed, lonely woman, wondering if this life was worth continuing.

I know I have loving family that I adore, and so many dear friends, and yes, that all is so important and so helpful and supportive, and I'm so grateful for you all. But at the end of the day, I would still be alone in my bed to face the music.

But when I lay my head down on the pillow at night, there is a man beside me who makes me certain I want to wake up the next day. He is the reason I'm strong. He is the reason I'm brave. He is my inspiration and he is the reason I can be "inspirational."

I won't say that without him, I am nothing. Don't get me wrong, in the best of times I can stand on my own two feet just fine. But I will say that in the worst of times, without him, I ain't "all that."

So, here's to my beloved Aitch. You make every day worth living. And for every compliment I receive, the credit is truly yours. I love you so very much.

Nose Envy

July 24, 2011, 11:04 a.m.

I miss my nose.

I've been so focused on adjusting to my "new look" that it hadn't hit me that hard, until yesterday.

We went to a screening of a movie and on the way, I found myself in the passenger seat of Paul's car staring out the window at the noses of all the people in the cars around us – big ones, little ones, pretty ones and not so much. I felt an emotion I don't like, something I avoid like the plague. I felt jealous. Jealousy is a dangerous thing, an ugly state of mind. It's bad ju-ju, a negative vibe. I don't worry much about following the Ten Commandments; I certainly take the name of Lord in vain plenty. But I always thought "Thou shalt not covet ..." was just plain good advice. Jealousy only wastes energy and deepens misery.

I've always believed that if you want what someone else has, instead of being jealous, try to figure out what you need to do for yourself to get the thing that will satisfy your desires, instead of wasting time wishing for what someone else has.

But this time I can't do that. There's nothing I can do to get a new nose. With patience, I'll eventually have a beautiful prosthetic. But I will never again have my own nose. A hard pill to swallow.

I'm grateful for my TFN, I truly am. Without it, I don't know how I'd get through the next three-to-six months. That said, it's not very comfortable, the condensation problem is unsolvable – I get water literally dripping out from under it – it draws way too much attention, and is just an all-around pain in the ass to wear.

I miss my nose. I miss looking like other people. I miss just answering the door without having to stick something on my face before I do.

And it's not just a visual thing. My face feels physically different without it, like something large is missing. And of course, there is. And I miss blowing it, wiping it, scratching it, picking it – and I don't even mean that to be funny, though I know it will get a laugh.

I know Paul misses my nose, too. Even though he's been wonderful. Even though he swears that as long as I'm there, he doesn't care about my nose. Still, it can't be easy to sit across the breakfast table from someone with a scooped-out face.

Even Bailey misses my nose. For 15 years, he's been licking my nose in what can only be described as a "mutual grooming" ritual he and I would share. I would pet a bunch of excess fur off of him and he would lick my nose thoroughly until I could no longer stand his sandpaper tongue. This saved me a lot of exfoliating. He and I have figured out a way to adjust. I offer him my chin instead, and he accepts it, but still, it's not the same.

I miss my nose.

It's that weird physical wrenching emptiness in the chest that grief produces. The feeling that was certainly the origin of the phrase "it broke my heart."

My heart has been broken many times. I've lost my parents, I've lost beloved pets, I've lost dear friends who died far too young. I've said Kaddish (the Jewish prayer of mourning) for all of them. But you can't really say Kaddish for a nose, so I'll just say RIP, dear nose. I will grieve you for a long, long time.

Today may be a good day to avoid mirrors.

A Tree Grows On Sixth Street

July 25, 2011, 11:26 a.m.

Once upon a time, OK, eight years ago to be specific, we moved into an upstairs duplex on Sixth Street. One of the attractions of the place was the many windows and abundant greenery.

Outside the master bedroom window was a particularly enormous tree. It was some kind of conifer that I have never been able to identify – a spruce perhaps? It towered above our duplex, creating shade and privacy for our bedroom, but still allowing a good view of the street. I loved lying on the bed where I could see the tree with its wide protective branches. We could easily see out, but others could not see in.

The tree was not just a haven for us. Over the years, many squirrels had made their homes there. We've seen a raccoon mom and baby and more than one possum come out of that tree in the dark of night. The longer we lived there, the more we loved that tree.

Fast forward about six years. One morning, our landlord informed us the tree would be cut down. It was leaning quite a bit and had become a danger, particularly to the house next door, and therefore, a liability.

Horrified, we begged to save the tree. Couldn't they just cut off the top part that was dangerous and leave the rest of the tree standing? Our landlord, a kind and caring man, agreed there was value in the tree and seeing what it meant to us, instructed the guys to do just that.

Unfortunately, the tree-trimmers were not artists – not even close. They hacked away at the upper branches, and finally just did a straight saw-off of the tree about 15 feet up – leaving a raw, ugly gaping wound.

It hurt to look at the tree where it had been cut. It oozed sap, as though attempting to heal itself. People say plants can feel things. If that is true, this tree must have been in agony. I wondered if it could even survive. But it did.

Still, there was little pleasure now in staring out at something so raw and ugly. I learned to guide my gaze downward, where the branches still grew thick and green.

Then, finally, more than a year later, a few little shoots began to grow, and little by little over the coming months, more signs of life appeared. But not enough. Never enough to cover the wound, to hide the pain.

Yesterday morning, alone in the house and engulfed in grief for my nose, I laid down on the bed where the cats were sleeping to try to soothe myself. I cried as I stretched out with a heavy heart, and as always, I eventually raised my eyes to the window.

I saw something then, something that so lifted me up that it brought me out of despair and back into the light. For the first time, I realized the new branches on the tree had finally grown large and high enough to completely cover the tree's giant wound. I rose from the bed and went to the window to look more closely. I knew the sawed-off edge was there, and if I looked very hard, I could still see it through the branches, but to all the rest of the world, no one would ever have known the tree had suffered such a trauma.

Our conifer looked whole again, beautiful and bountiful, with long, needled branches reaching out every which way. It wouldn't die, it would live, and probably for a very long, long time.

And so will I.

News, But Not Really

July 26, 2011, 10:30 p.m.

After an emotional weekend, today brought back a round of "cancer business," and some news – sort of. I'm learning that no news is ever really news because the actual things that determine the news are very fluid. Did y'all follow that? I'm not even sure I did, and I wrote it.

So, here's the latest: My surgeon spoke to the pathologist and they've determined the remaining microscopic melanoma in situ cells – above my lips below where my nose used to be – are actually not related to the original cancer. In other words, they are just random cells – not part of the desmoplastic tumor I lost my nose to.

This is great news because if it was part of the original cancer, I would absolutely, positively have to have more surgery and it would mean the really bad stuff had already spread and before it was all over, I'd be sporting a Phantom of the Opera mask. Yikes!

That said, here's the downside: in situ cells can become full-blown cancer at any time. This means that they can do more surgery – take a little bit of skin, check it out under the microscope and if they see more cells, take another little piece. The problem is, they could end up "chasing" the cells and take lots of my skin and never see the end of it. The other possibility is that they could take a piece, get clean margins and still not get it all because the cells can "jump" to another part of the face.

So, the consensus between two of my doctors is not to do surgery at this point, but to take a "wait and watch" approach, carefully monitoring me – forever. Then I had to get the melanoma specialist to weigh in, and that confused me even more, though ultimately, I think we're all on the same page now.

Finally, I still have the tumor board a week from Friday, and until I see them, and then do the follow-up with my surgeon, nothing is written in stone.

But at this point, I'm strongly leaning toward not doing surgery or radiation, because doing so would dramatically slow my path for my prosthesis. It's still a few months away since I have to completely heal before they can prepare it, but better a few months, than many.

That prosthesis is like a shining beacon off in the distance. It's the key to everything right now. This morning I was standing at the sink in front of the kitchen window and the Arrowhead guy came to the back porch to drop off our water bottles. I was about to knock on the window and wave, but then realized I didn't have my nose on! Can you imagine how freaked out he would have been? So instead, I ducked down below the counter so he couldn't see me.

That prosthesis means no more ducking below the kitchen counter! That prosthesis means I won't be Cancer Girl – or Bagel Face. My sister and I came up with that one today.

That prosthesis means no more staring children. That prosthesis means life as close to normal as I'm ever going to get again.

On a final note, I did take a big step today. I saw a client. She was referred to me and I happen to know she lost her husband to cancer, so she has more experience with it than anyone wants to. That made her a very safe person to start with. It was wonderful to be back up to my old tricks, holding my 25-foot Stanley tape measure in my fist, standing in an empty closet. But it was more exhausting than I imagined. Man, it takes a lot of energy to talk to strangers, think on your feet, be creative, answer questions and be gracious, warm and knowledgeable all at the same time! I feel kind of like Sampson after Delilah cut off all his hair, as though when they cut off my nose, I lost all my strength!

But I took that first step. And that felt like a pretty big deal. Now I need to sleep. Another doctor visit tomorrow.

It's endless.

You Haven't Changed A Bit

July 27, 2011, 8:51 p.m.

I do not ever go out in public without my TFN. However, a couple of dear friends with whom I feel safe have been brave enough to see me in all my holey-faced glory at home. Likewise, a few trusted friends and family who are far away have expressed a desire to know the "new" me, and I have obliged by sending them pictures.

What hadn't occurred to me, but nevertheless delighted me, is that I got the same response from all of them. They all said in one way or another: "I was so relieved to see it's still you."

It hadn't dawned on me that people were expecting me to be so changed that I would be unrecognizable. I was happy to hear them express that sentiment, of course, while at the same time not quite getting it, until tonight.

Paul and I were standing in the kitchen, and I was excited about something – I can't even remember what it was now – and made a face at him and gave him a big thumbs up. He suddenly gave me the widest grin that I could tell was unrelated to my own excitement.

"What?" I asked.

He said quite gently and sweetly, and with some relief, "Your face still has all the same expressions you've always had, and I can see them all, even without your nose." He then attempted to mimic a few of my vast repertoire of dramatic mugs, and I finally got it.

From inside of myself, it's me, it's always been me, it will always be me. From the outside, one might think missing a nose would alter that. Today's Life Lesson – Life seems to throw them at me with great regularity now.

The nose is just not that big a participant in how we express ourselves. It's all in the eyes and the mouth, isn't it? I never really took that apart before until Paul said it just that way.

What I'm really looking forward to and will really mean I've come full circle will be attending my 40th high school reunion next summer. By then, I hope to be all comfy and secure in my new prosthesis. I'm sure to bump into someone who won't know I've had cancer. I can't wait to hear them say, "Bunny Caplan, you haven't changed a bit!"

What a good laugh I'll have about that!

Herschel Caplan's Daughter
– The Flip Side

July 28, 2011, 7:03 p.m.

First, a joke. I had another chunk cut out of me today. A little lump on my upper arm that's probably nothing, but now every new blip must be biopsied, no matter how harmless it seems. The doctor said it would require a single stitch and with a look of great concern he told me that unfortunately, it would leave a scar.

I literally laughed in his face.

The doctor and nurse both looked shocked at my response.

Seriously? SERIOUSLY? You're worried about a quarter–inch scar on my arm that no one will ever see after they've just cut my nose off! I was laughing so hard, I couldn't speak. So, I just pointed to the giant mess in the middle of my face.

The lightbulb went off. They both got the joke, and suddenly Dr. Goldstein, the nurse, Paul and I were all loudly guffawing at the ridiculousness of it all.

And once again, I was told what a "great attitude" I have.

Everyone at Kaiser – doctors, nurses, physician's assistants, phlebotomists – a "look-it-up" word if ever there was one – keeps telling me how I have such a positive outlook, yada yada, and how that will help my healing.

I wrote recently about the pressure of being told I'm "inspiring" since I don't see myself that way. But I do admit to having some pride about my attitude.

So where did I get my upbeat view of life? Am I this way because of my parents or is it something inherent in who I am? The classic "nature vs. nurture" question. My wonderfully wise Sounding Board (Paul) concluded the answer is both, but we agreed the scales tip heavily in favor of my parents.

The irony here is that I do not believe either of my parents, individually, would have been able to deal with a disfiguring cancer and still keep a smile on their face.

Knowing both my parents, I'm guessing my father might have become bitter and angry. My mother, a woman to whom appearances were everything, would have felt humiliated and isolated. I say this not to denigrate either of them. They were both intelligent, gifted people. But neither of them had the benefit of something I did have. Neither had loving, supportive, nurturing parents.

I, on the other hand, was blessed and fortunate enough to have them as my parents. And they did something amazing. They rose above the example set by their own parents, who were all MIA, mostly for circumstances beyond anyone's control. My dad, especially, was always there for me, reading bedtime stories, tucking me in, willing to help me, give me a ride someplace, work on a school paper. There was nothing more wonderful than to be tucked inside my dad's arm while we watched TV together – "The Untouchables," "The Defenders," "Perry Mason." And he always knew "who done it" long before the end – a skill he passed along to me, much to my husband's annoyance.

My mother thought everything I did was miraculous. If I wrote a poem, it was the best poem ever! If I drew a picture, it was the best picture ever! And this was really a stretch, since art is clearly my sister's gift, not mine.

More than anything, they both showered me with love

and affection – sometimes to the point of overkill, I might add – but they raised me in an environment where I felt safe and secure and loved.

Add to that mix the fact that my sister actually wanted a little sister, begged my mother for one (so I'm told), and I got the benefit of having not one, but in a sense, two loving mother figures in my most formative years, before my sister grew into a teenager and decided I was just a little pain-in-the-butt, as any teenager in their right mind would.

So, this journal entry is a tribute to my father who taught me that being smart had value even though I was a girl, that reading and language are the keys to great thinking, and that I could do anything I set my mind to. And to my nurturing mother who set an example of treating others with kindness and passed on to me a great appreciation for the arts, and to my protective big sister – minus those few teen years.

Whenever I pick myself up, dust myself off and march forward with my chin held high, it's thanks to the three of them. And my loving husband, of course!

As sad as I am that I no longer have my parents around, in a way, I'm glad they're not here to see what I'm going through. They couldn't bear to see any of their children suffer, so I'm happy they were spared this. When all goes as it should in the so-called "Circle of Life," we must all bid our parents goodbye. But I'm ever so grateful that mine left me well-armed against the slings and arrows of outrageous fortune. I think my Dad would have liked ending with a Shakespearean reference.

Schlaf Gesunderheit, Herschel and Muriel.

The English Major Patient

July 30, 2011, 1:45 p.m.

Yesterday I was too busy living life to write about it. I think that's a good thing. I had one window in the day when the choice was between writing and resting, and resting won out.

But apparently it wasn't enough, because today I'm feeling it big time. No energy ... at ... all.

Of course, I was busy with good things (at least it wasn't doctor appointments). I actually saw a client in the morning. The universe was, once again, kind enough to send my way someone with whom I could feel comfortable – a referral that just happens to have run an oncologist's office and has seen it all. It's starting to get spooky (in a good way), how these clients are coming my way right now.

I am still not emotionally or physically ready to knock on the door of a complete stranger and deal with all the unknown factors involved. But in the meantime, I love being able to meet with "safe" people in a controlled way and not just sit around being a bump on a log (as my dad used to say). It makes me feel productive.

What made such a long day, though, was something very special. We had a visit from East Coast family, Paul's cousins. It was so good to see them and we had a wonderful time together. And they were gracious enough to cook a spectacular dinner for us where they are staying – which meant we could spend quality time together, but I wouldn't have to go sit in a busy restaurant on a Friday night.

Even as I write this, it's strikes me as completely bizarre that I would not want to sit in a busy restaurant on a Friday night. In my previous incarnation, I never shied away from busy places. I found them energizing and fun. And I didn't even have to be accompanied by anyone to enjoy them.

I was incredibly independent. Before I met Paul, I traveled alone, ate in restaurants alone and thought nothing of going to a movie alone. I enjoyed it, in fact. I held the belief then (and still do), that you have to be able to enjoy your own company in order to truly enjoy the company of others.

So, it's completely antithetical to my nature that I have become someone who avoids busy places and prefers to have a "shield" of another person in public. I'm hoping that feeling will dissipate over time. I feel so adjusted to life at home, I have to keep reminding myself that I've been through something life-altering that affects how I operate out in the world. I'm trying to be patient with myself.

Hmmm. For nearly three months now, I've been "a patient." Perhaps this is why those of us undergoing medical treatment are called that word? Because having a disease or an injury means you are constantly in waiting rooms of tardy doctors, or awaiting test results, and waiting – finally – to feel whole again?

Well, maybe it's just because I'm very worn out from yesterday's activity, but today I feel tired of being "patient." Three months is long enough. Is this mess over yet? Where's my new nose? I want my freedom back.

But of course, three months is a drop in the bucket, and the mess isn't over yet. I won't have my new nose probably for months. But I could have my freedom back. That is the one thing I could do. There is nothing actually stopping me. Except that I'm just not ready.

The oncology social worker tells me many people in my situation isolate and never leave the house, so she is pleased that I've been out as much as I have. I've taken plenty of baby steps. We go to our little neighborhood pizza joint or breakfast place. We go to the grocery or drug store. We go out for frozen yogurt. We go to the movies. I see safe clients. I have quiet lunches with girlfriends. But there are some things that still just feel too daunting.

So, I guess that means I'm still a "patient." And that's just the way it is – for now.

Is it 2012 yet?

Stuck in the Middle

July 31, 2011, 7:58 p.m.

Life goes on no matter what you are going through. Furry family members still need care, so today we took William in for a dental cleaning. Siamese cats are like the British; they have a reputation for lousy teeth.

He's never been anesthetized before, and now that we've brought him home with his sparkling pearly whites all in good order, he doesn't know what to do with himself. He's still in that semi-drugged state, but wide awake.

He's wandering around the house aimlessly. He sits. He gets up. He sniffs at something and then gets distracted. Noises make him jump. In other words, he's completely at loose ends.

I know exactly how he feels.

I'm back in that space myself today. I'm tired, but sick of resting. I don't want to lay down, but I don't have it in me to do anything much. I'm too tired to talk to people, but I don't want to be alone with my thoughts. Paul's taking a well-deserved nap, so I'm left to my own devices. I'm sick to death of random TV, and I don't have the focus to read.

I'm fine when I have a purpose or a task. I'm also fine when I'm exhausted and taking a snooze. It's this "in the middle" thing I can't stand. Awake, but feeling inert.

This journal entry seems quite whiny to me, but hey, it's how I feel. Whiny. Can't you just hear the little kid in me screaming: "But I don't wanna have cancer." (Insert vision of my lower lip sticking out and the toe of my shoe kicking the dirt).

Tomorrow will begin a new week, and I'll have new

distractions of a few clients and a lot of doctors, so I'm sure the feeling will pass.

In the meantime, maybe I'll just shadow Big William around the house and the two of us can be at loose ends together. It's always comforting to be in the presence of our furry beasts.

Wherever he hangs out, I think I'll hang out too. If he stretches out on the cool linoleum in the kitchen, I'll stretch out right beside him. If he pauses on the couch to stare out the window, so will I. But let me just say straight up, if he starts to lick his butt, well, that's where I'll have to draw the line!

Birds Do It, Bees Do It, Even Girls with the Big C Do It

August 1, 2011, 10:24 p.m.

If I'm going to be real, I'm going to be really real. Nothing kicks the Cancer Blues' ass like finally having a "date" (wink wink) with your husband.

I confess this was a scary proposition for so many reasons. There were the obvious concerns: Can I get my head in the right space? How will my body respond after coming through surgery? Will I have the energy to enjoy it? And of course the $64,000 question: Just how sexy can a gal be with no nose?

The answer: Apparently, sexy enough!

Perhaps even more intimate than the experience itself, was the discussion that followed in which we admitted all our worries.

You'd think after 15 years with my amazing Aitch that I'd take for granted we'd be on the same page with this, but still, it was a huge relief to find out he was as concerned as I was – about different things perhaps – but I am so happy and thankful that we draw strength from each other to fight the fear and move past it.

Of all the things I've lost with my cancer diagnosis, not the least of which is my nose, to add "loss of consortium" (as they say in the legal field) to the list would have been the straw that most certainly would have broken this camel's back.

But I needn't have worried. Today, another hurdle was conquered in the aftermath of this daunting disease. Little by little, in bits and pieces, normal does return.

On a completely different note: My other great joy of the day? Paul's iPod has been acting up and this evening I fixed it for him. After being cared for by this man for weeks on end and feeling helpless and useless, it absolutely tickled me pink to do something for him for a change!

Today was a good day!

Ch-ch-ch-ch-changes, Turn and face the strain

August 3, 2011, 10:08 p.m.

Well, I had to pull David Bowie out of the hat sooner or later. I'm from that generation. This song always seemed to fit whatever in my life was happening. Probably because life is always changing. Hell, life is change.

I always try to remember that no matter how bad things get, and no matter how good things are, the one thing you know for sure is that eventually things will change.

That said, I wrote a while back that this whole "cancer thing" wouldn't change me, that if anything, I would grow from it, not shrink from it. That's only partly true.

Last night I had dinner with a very dear old friend who suffered the tragic loss of her daughter a few years ago. She said she spent quite some time declaring loudly how she would not let it change her. But last night she shrugged, shook her head and said, "I finally realized that's crazy. Of course it changed me. How could it not?"

Boy, did that hit a nerve.

Then, before bed last night I was reading a book, a gift from my friend, Joy, by Luis Montalvan, a former soldier, about his service dog who helps him cope with PTSD and other injuries he sustained in Iraq. Montalvan says: "You're a changed person after combat. Not better or worse, just different. Seeking or wishing for the old you are the worst thing you can do." Switch out "combat" for "cancer" – same difference. There's a reason the expression is "she's battling cancer."

Once again, hit the same nerve. Same message from two different places on the same night. When this happens, I always believe the universe is trying to tell me something.

It took me awhile, but tonight I figured out a little piece of it, though I suspect I'll be learning this particular lesson for months to come.

But here was the light bulb:

Another friend asked me tonight why I didn't think I could return to work, when I look pretty OK with my temporary fake nose.

No one had asked me this question point blank, and until now I have not been able to articulate why I'm not ready to knock on the door of an absolute stranger and put myself in a completely uncontrolled situation.

But as I tried to explain it to him, I finally got clear on it.

Most clients are fine. Many are fun, interesting, nice people. But there are those few that are not. They are disrespectful, demeaning, negative and some are downright crazy. Though it's rare, there are clients who have completely unnerved me – and that can happen when I'm at my best and strongest.

It would only take one person, one crazy asshole, to say something insensitive or mean, and I would be completely undone. I am so emotionally fragile right now, there is no way on the planet that I would bounce right back from an encounter with the wrong kind of client. I have a hard enough time dealing with well-meaning questions from strangers on the street – and I can turn on my heel and walk away from them if I want!

Sure, my journal entries may make it sound like I'm all strong and brave and blah blah blah, but that's in the presence of people who love me and care about me. As long as I feel safe, I'm Barbara the Lion-Hearted. But put me in an uncontrolled environment alone without Paul or a friend as a buffer, and watch me whither.

Don't get me wrong. I know this is perfectly normal. I know that I'm actually doing "better than the average bear" when it comes to getting out and about. I also know the fragility will lessen with time and certainly dissipate with the security of my actual prosthesis.

But it's finally sinking in that I am permanently altered, not just physically, but emotionally as well. I will never again feel invincible. One stupid little dark spot and my nose is gone and my life expectancy statistically shortened. My mortality is real, palpable. It's just another little freckle away.

So yes, I admit it. I accept it. I am changed. And therein lies the paradox, because I'm also still just me!

A Little Slice of Heaven

August 4, 2011, 8:40 p.m.

It's days like today that give me strength and keep me going.

Two people who know me from two completely different arenas of my life, both referred me recently to a place called WeSpark Cancer Support Center. Thank you, Kathrin and Lauren. And if you read yesterday's journal entry, you know what I think about getting the same message from two different places!

So today I decided to go. I did an intake session with a wonderful, compassionate woman named Bonnie. We spent over an hour talking and then she explained all the things the center has to offer. They have yoga, Pilates, tai chi, guided imagery, writing workshops, support groups for cancer patients in varying stages of treatment – and even mah jong classes!

Better still, they have individual body work – Reiki, Qi Gong, hypnotherapy and all sorts of other healing stuff.

And it's all FREE! Well, sort of. There is a tiny little price. You or a family member must have cancer in order to utilize their services. I know, I know. Some people will do anything to get free body work.

After my intake with Bonnie, there just happened to be a cancellation with an amazing Reiki and massage therapist who is otherwise booked for weeks in advance. Woohoo! A lucky break, indeed.

I have very little experience with Reiki, but an interesting thing happened. When the session began, I felt this enormous desire to take big, long, deep breaths. I am not a person who is naturally inclined to deep breathing. All those years I spent dancing, teachers were constantly yelling at me – "keep breathing!"

But in the hands of this woman, Debbie, breathing deeply and calmly felt like the most natural thing in the world. It was only when the session was over and we were talking about it that I realized how physically closed off I had become these past few months. When you are under-going treatment for cancer – or any illness for that matter – you are constantly being prodded, poked and peered at, and your body just wants to close in on itself as a defense against the pain and invasion of things being done to you.

Most amazing of all was this: While Debbie was working on my feet, I suddenly felt the presence of my mother. It was emotional and overwhelming, and I don't understand how or why, but I felt her in the room with us. Debbie told me later that everyone responds to Reiki differently, but that she has had other patients who have felt the presence of a lost loved one.

I know there are some of you out there who will pooh-pooh this, and guess what? I don't care! Explain it any way you'd like. Chalk it up to emotional stress. But I felt her there with me. It was only for a moment, but it was powerful.

At the end of my three hours there, I felt renewed in a way I haven't felt since we left Yosemite in May. Relaxed, relieved and open.

So that's how I spent my afternoon – in a place with a most incredible healing energy that is palpable when you walk in the door. Talk about a safe environment! If only it could last.

But tomorrow …

… tomorrow I face the tumor board. I'm terrified they are going to tell me radiation is the only way to get "clean."

Four hours with multiple doctors in my face (literally). I have no idea what state of mind I will be in after it's over.

But I am glad I at least got today. One day of utter peace.

Gratitude and Celebration!

August 5, 2011, 9:43 p.m.

FINALLY! I'm thrilled to announce the doctors agree. There isn't any great benefit from my having radiation therapy.

First, the melanoma in situ cells that are still there are in what's called a "wide field," i.e., who knows where they all are on my face. And they don't want to just radiate my whole face. In essence, it has the same problem as surgery. How do you go "chasing" microscopic cells and ever be certain you got them all?

As many of you know, once you have radiated a spot, you have greatly diminished healing capacity for future surgery (not to mention all the other possible side effects). This is too high a price to pay and still not be sure you've gotten it all.

And yes, I have a chance of recurrence, but radiation wouldn't reduce those odds, it would only impact a new melanoma developing from the existing in situ cells.

Finally, and most salient I think, is the fact that there is great disagreement about the percentage of in situ cells that actually become malignant cancer. The range is five percent – 30 percent. Still, even going by the most conservative numbers, 70 percent of in situ cells do NOT become malignant.

The third option, which everyone agrees is the best, is to take a "wait and watch" approach. I will, for the rest of my life, be seeing a dermatologist on a very regular basis. The doctors say that Paul and I are actually going to be the most important factors in catching something new, because we are most likely to see something when it appears.

And it will be my job to show up to the doc for every new little spot or bump. That's a job I can do, and happily so!

It was quite an experience of having four doctors look at me at once, taking turns feeling my neck and head, and then all four observing while they put a scope down my "cavity" to make sure there was no nasty cancer lurking where no one had looked.

Perhaps the weirdest thing about the whole day was that the original radiologist we met with this morning had actually seen my nose post-surgery! He had been with the pathologist when he was working on it and saw it intact after they had removed it from my face and before they sliced and diced it for the pathology report.

He thought then what an interesting case it was, so he was stoked that he actually got to meet with me. How bizarre is that!?! But it made me feel a strange bond with him – it's like how you feel about the person who was the last to see a loved one alive. They are your final connection to the loved one. It was kind of bittersweet meeting him, like – "oh, he knew my nose."

Anyway, it was an early morning and a long, exhausting day, but it's over!

On Wednesday, I'll see my surgeon and get a better idea of how short (or long) the wait will be before I'm ready to meet again with the prosthodontist about starting work on my new nose.

In the meantime, my surgical site continues to heal and actually shrink (a good thing), which allowed me to trim my TFN so it's a bit more comfortable than it had been. It's still a pain-in-the-face, but I feel like I can at least see a bit better now, as I was able to pare down the area between my eyes.

Progress in bits and pieces. Now it's about getting my energy back and regaining my emotional health and strength so I can start to face the world again with confidence.

On a final note, the other weird thing today was a little revelation I had this morning. The line to check-in to see the doctors was long. Because it's the home of all the radiation and chemo work for Kaiser, many people in line wore hats, or wigs and had obviously lost their hair. I scanned the group and felt a sad little tug at my heart. All these poor people had cancer, so sad. Then I realized, I'm in this line! I have my hair, but I don't have my nose. I am one of "those poor people."

I guess my autopilot consciousness just hasn't fully assimilated it yet, but it will. The treatment portion of this journey is over, but once you have cancer, it's never completely absent from your life. My big task now is to learn to live with the uncertainty of recurrence, and be able to let go of that fear.

In the meantime, I'm going to sip some champagne with my Aitch to end the long day. I'm guessing I'll be sleeping my way through most of tomorrow! But that's OK. It'll be restful sleep, not "avoidance sleep." What a nice change!

Top Ten Things
I'm Grateful For

August 7, 2011, 1:46 p.m.

I'm still floating from Friday's good news that I will not need further treatment. I'm grateful for so many things, but here's my Top Ten List in no particular order (all have been mentioned in previous posts, but they bear repeating now):

1.) The brilliant dermapathologist who discovered a difficult to diagnose cancer before it metastasized, thus saving my life.

2.) Amazing health coverage, so what might have meant financial ruin, has only meant "let's tighten belts and find a way through this."

3.) Supportive and patient bosses, (Jose, John, Mary), including our owner (Mr. Melkonian), who have allayed any concerns about losing my job, insurance, or their respect, while I go through this difficult experience. I can't thank them enough!

4.) Caring Bridge, my lifeline to everyone, and through which I've been bolstered daily by so many kind notes. And it's been quite therapeutic to look inside every day, examine what's happening to me, and have a place where I can give voice to those thoughts and feelings.

5.) My compassionate doctors and nurses, none of whom made me feel stupid or bothersome as I bombarded them with questions. I always felt in control of my treatment, that choices were mine, but all were willing to give me information I needed to make good decisions.

6.) My friends and family who have all been stellar.

Thanks especially to DeeDee and Sara, and to my BFF's: Vicky, Jami, Barbara, Nancy, Kathrin, Tara, to name a few. Special mention goes to my high school sweetheart (now dear friend), Dr. Steve Denenberg. His assistance with medical issues and research was invaluable. I so appreciate the time he spent arming with me all the right questions.

7.) My "boyz," William and Bailey, who make me smile every single day no matter what, and who don't give a rat's ass what I look like ever.

8.) That I only lost my nose. You heard me. I only lost my nose. Some people lose so much more to melanoma — large portions of their jaw, teeth, eyes — all things that have a profound impact on one's ability to eat, see, smell, taste. All I lost was a measly skeletal shell with mucous and hair inside. (Gee, when you put it that way.)

9.) It may sound weird, but I'm grateful that I am who I am. I don't take credit for this. I've always been lucky. And while I do believe we make our own luck, that's only part of the story. Shit does happen. And I've been extraordinarily fortunate throughout my entire life in how the things I can't control have somehow gone my way.

10.) Finally — saving the best for the last — you've heard it all ad nauseam, but I am most grateful to my incredible husband, to my Paul, my Aitch, the Love of My Life, the man who has been all I could ask for and so much more throughout this entire ordeal. He has made me feel beautiful, even when looking in the mirror says everything to the contrary.

He has never made me feel, even for a second, that he would ever not be at my side, no matter what. He has taken care of me, kept me laughing, let me cry when I needed to, and so much more. Without him, well, I don't even want to contemplate that. I don't know if I'll be posting daily anymore. The journey isn't over, but the pace is slowing down.

If you don't want to have to check this space every day, you can sign up for email notification for when I do post.

I know many people have been talking about a book from all this. I am a writer, which means I know you don't write the book while you're still in the middle of the story. So that will be something to work on down the road, when I've gained some perspective. But I appreciate all the encouragement!

And now, on to the prosthesis! Stay tuned.

The Little Engine That Still Couldn't

August 8, 2011, 9:54 p.m.

Very short note tonight to beg everyone's indulgence. I owe so many emails and phone calls, and there are so many people to whom I owe thank you's for all the amazing ways they've found to support me.

These are calls and notes I want to make, but am finding it nearly impossible to garner the energy to do it, except in drips and drabs ... an email here, a phone call there.

It's very deceptive, because when I'm fine, I'm fine! I feel like myself and like I'm supposed to be able to conquer the world.

In those first couple of weeks after surgery, I had full license to be silent on all fronts. But now that I'm better, I feel that permission to be nonresponsive slipping away. I tend to forget that I'm still recuperating. What happens, unfortunately, is that I will run out of steam very suddenly and without warning. Like now ...

For those of you expecting to hear from me but have not, thanks for your patience. I'll get there eventually!

But now, it's only 8 p.m. and all I want to do is crawl into bed. Since cats sleep 80 percent of the day, I'm always guaranteed good company!

Too Tired For a Clever Title

August 10, 2011, 11:59 p.m.

First, I want to pay a special tribute to a woman I have never met but developed a great admiration for. Janine Millar–Sax lost her battle with cancer yesterday. She fought long and hard, and her husband, Jeff – a friend of Paul's – was her champion and caregiver who stuck by her side through every rough moment and did it all with adoration and love. Even while he was going through his own difficult journey, Jeff always offered a supportive shoulder to Paul as he traveled this road with me. My heart breaks for him tonight, and I wanted to honor Janine with a special mention of her here. She was a bright spirit and I'm so sorry she is gone.

I'm too tired again to write much but wanted to offer a brief update. Saw my surgeon today. My healing is going well with the exception of a couple of tiny spots where a stitch never dissolved and where the grafted skin isn't quite heal-ing over the bone yet, but we are keeping an eye on those and they should be fine. No big deal. Overall, he thought my rate of healing was extraordinary.

I did ask about my continued lack of energy. He kind of smiled like, "Are you crazy?" He then patiently told me that my body is using an enormous amount of energy to try to heal the giant wound in my face. On top of that, anyone who's been told they have cancer and must lose a body part suffers from a certain form of post–traumatic stress (not exactly the same as soldiers, but a variation on that theme).

He was not at all surprised at my inability to "go all day" like I used to.

Of course, many people have said this, not the least of which is Paul, but I guess I had to hear it from the doctor. Now I can let myself be and not feel like I'm being a big baby or over-indulgent.

The doc was also pleased that I'm seeing a few repeat clients and thought my inability to see new clients yet was not at all unexpected. He said, "I'd worry about you if you said you were fine and ready to do it all. You'd be in serious denial and headed for a fall." I'm paraphrasing here, but you get the idea.

It's all good. I was kind of hoping he would tell me I'm ready to head off to UCLA for my prosthesis, but I have a lot more healing to do. I'll be seeing them at the end of September to see if they think I'm ready to start the process then. It's just so difficult to predict the rate of healing.

Finally, I had a Qi Gong session today at WeSpark. It's a healing energy thing. A fascinating experience. I was a bit skeptical at first, but when it was over, I did feel a great release of stress energy that I'd been holding in. I'm trying to be open to anything that helps relieve fear and stress and promotes healing. Next week: reflexology!

Phantom of the Nostril

August 12, 2011, 8:51 p.m.

At least once a night, I wake up with a wild itching, usually just inside my left nostril and I reach up to scratch. My finger hits empty space and I remember – oh, yeah.

It reminds me of the feeling I had after we lost our beloved Siamese, Amanda, to cancer. She used to sleep curled up against me, and if I awoke from a weird dream, I'd automatically reach out to pet her. For months after she died, if I awoke in the middle of the night, I'd still put my hand out to touch her, but it would hit empty space – just like now – and I would feel that terrible grieving ache with the realization she was gone.

But unlike my experience with Amanda, this "phantom itch" happens at least half a dozen times throughout my waking hours as well. Every single time I will reach up to scratch a nose that isn't there. It's been over five weeks, and the automatic response is strong as ever. It's maddening to have an itch you can't scratch, and a little bit funny because it's so damn weird, and more than a little sad because of what it means: "Oh yeah, I have no nose."

At first, I would get upset when it happened because it would make me miss my nose. But it happens so often now that I've worn out my emotional response, desensitized myself in a way. Although I still react with great annoyance every time because it drives me crazy!

Probably everyone has heard of phantom pain or itching for people who have had a limb amputated, but I never dreamed it would happen with a nose! I'm told it can last a few months, a few years, or the rest of my life.

What's interesting to me is that we all know grief is an emotion – we feel something in our proverbial "hearts." Phantom sensations, though, are a physiological response. So in essence, it's like the body itself grieves for what it lost. I do believe the mind and body are one, and perhaps this is some kind of evidence of that?

I will always love and miss Amanda, but it's been over five years since she died, and I don't reach for her in my sleep anymore. I'm crossing my fingers that in five years, I won't still be reaching to scratch my absent nose.

And even if I do still feel the itch, I may not be able to reach to scratch, because after five years it will have driven me completely mad and I'll be wearing a straight-jacket!

Ah, what's a Friday night without a little melodrama?

What Happens in Vegas

August 13, 2011, 5:34 p.m.

Today, walking home from Yogurtland – it's my incentive for getting out of the house on a beautiful day – Paul and I were talking about how exhausted he is. We both are, but my reasons are obvious.

We both slept well last night. Both cats were mercifully quiet the entire night, and yet Paul was wondering why he's still so tired. My answer is this: We've been dancing as hard and as fast as we can for two months now, constantly making decisions, running to doctors, dealing with wound care, etc. For me, add the healing process; for him add the caretaking of me and running the household single-handedly.

And now, we're finally able to sit down and take a breath. That's when the weariness really hits you, I think.

So we're taking a break. We're gettin' outta Dodge. Packin' up the old jalopy. Hittin' the road, Jack. Headin' out on the highway. Feel free to fill in your favorite traveling cliché here.

We've got a free place to stay in Vegas, so that's where we're going. And I, the great worshipper of heat, will get a chance to bake in the shade and dip in the pool (TFN above water). Paul will play a little blackjack and read. We'll hit the cheap buffet at Southpoint Casino whenever we're hungry and that's about it!

We've done Vegas enough so that we won't feel compelled to do and see things. We can literally just kick back completely and utterly and totally.

No cats, no birds, no phone!

I know what happens in Vegas is supposed to stay in

Vegas, but I'd like the sense of relief and renewal that I'm hoping we achieve in those few days to last until we make it back to L.A. In other words, I hope what happens in Vegas doesn't stay in Vegas.

But first, gotta get through this next week.

Me and The Dow Jones

August 16, 2011, 9:50 p.m.

My mother had an expression that's apropos for the space I'm in: "I don't know whether I'm coming or going."

All last week, I was flying high on the news that radiation was not recommended. But in the cancer game, once you get over one hurdle, there just might be another one on the horizon.

Let me preface this by saying the worst is absolutely over, and I feel great about that. But now there are other issues – smaller issues – and fears creeping in, and for some reason, I've come crashing down from my high.

Let's start with my lip. As the surgical site shrinks and heals, it's started to asymmetrically lift one side of my Cupid's Bow – the double peaks of my lips – so that my lips are crooked – and not in a "cute" way. I thought I'd made my bargain with the cancer devil: Take my nose, but don't fuck with my smile! Apparently, the cancer devil is not good at keeping bargains.

My surgeon told me to pull on it to stretch the skin, but since he is an oncologist and not a plastic surgeon, I thought a call was in order to my dear friend, Steve, who is a plastic surgeon. And though he was dubious about the efficacy of "stretching" the skin, he did give me some reason to have hope that it might drop back down as the scar tissue softens. Still, it freaks me out to think the changes in my face are still not over. And thus began the spiral downward. Fragile psyches don't do well with surprises of this sort.

Then, for some reason, I've also started to stress out about whether or not I will qualify for having the Cadillac of prostheses, i.e., the nose that's held on by magnets. My bone density has to be sufficient (questionable) and other things about the site have to be in order. And even if I do qualify medically, will Kaiser cover the more expensive nose? Unknown and unknowable at this time.

So here we are back to the waiting game again. My appointment at UCLA isn't until September 20th, and that was me rushing it, because they won't start anything until the wound is fully healed, which may not be until sometime in October. But we'll see.

Anyway, I've been up and down so many times over the past few months that if I were a stock, you probably should have sold me back in the spring!

As I said to Paul, I just wish I could either jump back a year in time or forward a year in time. In his typical wisdom, he reminded me that going back is not an option, and going forward will happen, just a little slower than I'd like. Damn, that guy is just full of good come backs!

At least today was a self-care day. I had reflexology at WeSpark this morning, which was wonderful, and finally got my hair cut this afternoon, so I feel a little better.

But still, I'm just frickin' tired of and frustrated with the stupid TFN. It was fine to get me through a couple of weeks, but the thought of wearing it another few months is just bloody depressing.

I know, I know. It could be so much worse. And you all know from most of my posts how grateful I am about that. I'm just having a little pity party today.

Maybe it's PMS. You wouldn't think a woman my age would even be able to say that, but oh yes, I still can. My menopause seems to have gotten stuck on the "meno" and forgotten about the "pause."

TMI, guys? Sorry. You know I'm nothing if not real

on this site. You take your chances when you click on this link.

OK, enough moping. There is one thing, one beacon I've got my eye on right now. VEGAS, BABY! Give me that beautiful suite, the jacuzzi tub right in the room, the cheap buffet, and all the lounge chairs, heat and movies – there's a theatre on site – at my fingertips. We literally don't even ever have to get in the car, except that I will to go to the outlet mall!

Is it next week, yet? Better still, is it next year yet?

Whistle a Happy Tune

August 18, 2011, 10:18 a.m.

I love to whistle. I'm good at it. I often "whistle while I work," especially while measuring a closet. It's usually a reflection of the chipper mood I'm in and I sometimes do it quite unconsciously – much to my father's annoyance when I lived at home. He had the weird idea that whistling was unladylike. This from a pre-feminist era feminist!

Among the many odd and sad little discoveries I've made over the past few weeks, one of them was that I had lost my ability to whistle. I learned this when attempting to call William for his treats. I have a special whistle that he always comes to. But when I tried to pucker up, I realized that the edge of the skin graft was too tight to allow my upper lip to form a "proper pucker" – say that ten times fast! It's the same tightness that's making my lips asymmetrical.

This was horribly depressing.

Well, in the past few days, I've realized that getting my whistle back is a matter of "exercising." The more I work at it, the easier it becomes, though it's still far from what it was. It's like stretching muscles that have become tight from inactivity. Slowly, but I'm hoping surely, it will come all the way back. I can't imagine not ever being able to "Whistle a Happy Tune" again.

While we are on the subject of weird discoveries, since my surgery, I've had this weird feeling, like I want to "flare my nostrils," especially when I get a phantom itch, but I can't. One might say the reasons for this are obvious – I have no nostrils. But still, it felt like something was frozen that shouldn't be. In fact, the whole area in the middle of my face has felt like a giant black hole with no feeling and no connection to the rest of me, which is very disconcerting.

Well, again in the past few days, I've found the "flaring" muscle! I got the strangest sensation and worked at it and worked at it, until lo and behold, I wiggled the area of the skin graft where the bottom of my nose was! I know this sounds bizarre, but I can't tell you how exciting this was.

And at first, I could only do it intermittently. I would actually "lose" the muscle back into the numbness. So freaky! But now, I can do it at will every single time.

Physiologically speaking, I'm not sure how, if at all, the whistling and the wiggling are connected (it makes sense to me that they are besides the fact that they are alliterative), but it gives me hope that, as the tissue grows and repairs, and as the nerves and muscles all reestablish themselves, the giant, numb space in my face will eventually feel like part of my own body again and not like something foreign landed between my eyes and my mouth.

And this, in turn, proves my friend's point. Kathrin, a cancer survivor herself, said the changes in the scar tissue would be ongoing. This is key, because it means I won't be stuck where I am or where I've been. Maybe someday, I'll be wildly whistling and wiggling away, with my lips back to their symmetrical beauty, and I'll look back on all this as just a nasty blip in my life.

I guess this whole thing is constantly evolving. Hey, I'm evolutionary! But please don't tell the Creationists in Kansas, they may try to have me outlawed! (Ooh, political sass – I must be feeling better!)

And now, it's back to the Kaiser lab so the vampire phlebotomists can take more of my blood.

A Few of My Favorite Things

August 21, 2011, 10:50 a.m.

When faced with a potentially life-threatening illness, the finite nature of our time on this planet becomes all too real, and one tends to think about roads not traveled and ambitions unrealized. Since I don't know how much time I have left – none of us do, after all – what do I want to do with that time?

Once Paul and I felt the great relief of knowing the melanoma had not metastasized, but also being faced with the risk of recurrence, we had a talk about this and decided we would each come up with a short list of "must-do" things. For some reason, I don't like the name "bucket list." Then I met the gentleman at WeSpark who did Qi Gong on me. His name is Ed Sullivan. I know, I know. Paul has made more than one "really great shew" joke, and I can't say his name without bursting into the song from "Bye, Bye Birdie." But Ed suggested the very same thing – that I make just such a list to get clear on my priorities. He felt it would help me heal and move beyond my recent trauma.

Paul and I decided this would make a great topic of conversation for the ride to Vegas. Paul, of course, is already done with his list.

I have been thinking and thinking but haven't actually nailed anything down. It's odd to me that I couldn't do this simple exercise, until I finally realized why. Ask me what's my favorite movie. I'm dumbstruck. Gee, is it "Gone with the Wind?" "When Harry Met Sally?" "The Wizard of Oz?" "The Lord of the Rings" Trilogy? Anything by Hitchcock, or anything starring Cary Grant? How can I pick a favorite? They're all brilliant and so different, except that I still maintain "Lord of the Rings" pays strong homage to the symbolism and structure of "The Wizard of Oz," but that's a discussion for another place and time.

Same thing with authors. How could I possibly choose between Charlotte Bronte and John Irving? Between Mark Twain and Alice Hoffman? All brilliant, but so different. That game, pick three books you'd take if you knew you were going to be stranded on a desert island? Forget it!

I don't even have one favorite color, I have three – blue, green and yellow.

Perhaps this is my Gemini nature, not that I put much stock in astrology. I am a person of duality, and therefore have a hard time picking one thing out of many.

So how can I choose a few things to do before I die out of an endless list of possibilities? Some of what I do will be based on opportunity, and how can I possibly predict what doors might open for me in the years to come?

My other obstacle here is that I once did have a "must do" list, and I've done those things. I've seen my name in print more than once, I've written not one novel, but three (the "must do" list didn't say they had to be good!), I've traveled to England (more than once), which was at the top of my list of desires when I was younger.

Other than that, I've never been a person of great vision in that way. When I was a teenager, I never planned my wedding. I never had a picture of what my life would be like, where I would live, what I would do. Seriously. I thought choices would just become obvious when it was time to make them.

My ambitions were always more vague: Be a good person. Be respected. Be responsible. Help animals. Have adventures. Have fun. Laugh a lot. Be smart. Be a good mate to someone.

As I write this, I see that my ambitions were about ways to be, not things to do.

And yet, Paul and I do a lot. We travel somewhere new every year. We attend concerts, plays, events, we socialize, we volunteer – we do things. In fact, we joke that we are people who would rather do things than have stuff. We'd rather spend our money going places, having experiences and doing things than buying a new couch or a big flat-screen TV.

To boil it all down: There are several reasons I'm having trouble with this short list. First, I have a hard time narrowing down my choices on anything. Second, I've already done some of the important things I wanted to do. Finally, we do a lot already! See? I can't even pick one reason why I can't make a list!

I have less than 24 hours to come up with my list now and I'm no closer than I was two weeks ago. It isn't exactly "Sophie's Choice," a book that would certainly be on my lengthy list of favorite novels, but it is a serious challenge for a woman who is never able to pick just one favorite thing.

With one exception, of course. There is one very easy, very simple answer when asked who is the Love of My Life, my favorite man among men. I'd offer a prize to the person who can guess it, but anyone who's read more than one or two of these posts will know the answer.

A clue: Think of the letter between G and I. Now, where's some paper and a pen. I'm running out of time.

We Can Run,
But We Can't Hide

August 27, 2011, 10:58 p.m.

Well, we're back from Vegas, and other than the 116-degree heat (seriously!), it was a fine trip. We didn't do much, exactly as we planned. I read, laid by the pool when there was enough shade, ate a lot, played the slot machines (won a little, lost a little), and made a killing at the outlet mall (three lace tank tops for just $9.99 and $10 bras!).

The week brought several discoveries and realizations.

First, going to Vegas meant throwing myself into the public eye in a way I hadn't really thought much about in advance. It was OK because I was surrounded by complete strangers and could walk away from any situation that felt uncomfortable.

I got stared at – a lot. At the pool, in the casinos, walking on the strip, pretty much everywhere. I didn't really seem to care much, so I thought. I learned that if you smile at people, you put them at ease, and they smile back. I actually forgot sometimes that I have this big bandage on my face when I would make a casual comment to someone in a store or restaurant or casino. Then I would see how some of them would look at me and I would remember. Oh yeah, it's not just "me," it's "me and the bloody TFN!"

One bright spot was a little girl I crossed paths with in the ladies' room. She saw me and smiled and stuck out a foot. "Look at my shoes!" she commanded. I told her they were very nice shoes. Her next declaration was: "I like your

nose!" Her mother looked embarrassed, but I laughed and thanked her. Then she ordered, "Look at my dress!" At that point, her mother rolled her eyes and pulled her little one out through the door. But it was nice to have my nose admired between her boasts about her dress and shoes.
I believe the stickers I wore that day were a flower and a butterfly. Obviously, a winning combination to a three-year-old.

But despite that brief moment, I found my spirits sinking as the week wore on. I'm not one to hang out in my room, no matter how nice it is. Even if I want to relax and read, I prefer to sit poolside or somewhere outdoors. Leaving my room meant dealing with my TFN and facing humanity. Every day. For hours on end. I wore my TFN more in those few days than I ever had at home.

It took me until Thursday to figure out why I was depressed despite "getting away." It became clear when I woke up and looked in the mirror at the black void in the center of my face and had to cut myself a new dressing for the TFN.
I can leave town, but I can't "get away" from what I most wish to escape. And neither can Paul, because after all, this was supposed to be his "get away" too.

It doesn't matter where I go, because wherever I go, there I am. I can't escape my own face. I've never even wanted to before, so no wonder it took me awhile to figure it out.

It's been well over two months since the very first Mohs procedure on June 13. That morning was the last time I was able to look in the mirror see myself whole.

I know there is an end to this. I know the prosthesis will make things so much better. But I'm so far in and still have so far to go.

Tonight, I'm exhausted, and tonight, I'm sad.

I'm exhausted because it takes so much energy to be out in the public eye, but I just can't be a recluse. I just can't. It's completely antithetical to who I am. I have to dig deep for the energy and the strength.

Next weekend will bring the beginning of a three-week onslaught of out-of-town visitors coming from NYC, Minnesota, Florida and even British Columbia. Fortunately, they are all dear friends and family who I love and am eager to see. I'm hoping these visits will be a nice diversion in a way that Vegas wasn't. It will certainly be a wonderful way to lift my spirits.

And when the last visitor has gone, voila', it will be time for my appointment with the UCLA prosthodontist, and at least I'll feel like I'm taking a step forward. And as I've come to realize, treading water equals depression. Moving forward brings relief.

But the real discovery of the week is this: Whether I stand still or charge ahead, what's happening to me is inescapable, so why waste energy trying to run, when I really can't hide? It's as simple as that.

So What, I'm Still a Rock Star

August 30, 2011, 10:11 p.m.

I know "So What" by Pink is about kicking her husband out, which I have absolutely no intention of doing – EVER! In fact, thanks to my incredibly hip Aitch for introducing me to this song. But if you substitute cancer for husband, it's actually quite fitting. After my depression of the past few days, I found myself singing this song on the way into Kaiser to have my yearly check-up with my OB/GYN doc. Just because one has cancer doesn't mean one can let the rest of their health go to hell in a hand basket!

So there I was, walking to Kaiser, singing ...

> *"So what! I'm still a rock star,*
> *I got my rock moves,*
> *and I don't need you!"*

There's more good lyrics, but you get the picture. I'm all ready to rise back to the "fuck you, cancer" place I prefer to live.

Until I sit down with my doc and she tells me she wants to do an endometrial biopsy. Boom! I come crashing down faster than a pregnant pole-vaulter.

This is not really a big deal. It's precautionary because, as I mentioned earlier, my menopause has lost its "pause," which they have to make sure isn't something "dangerous."

Now, I have not had a meltdown in a doctor's office since the day I was told I should have the rhinectomy. But I did today. Somehow, after all I've been through, the idea of another test, another form of cancer, another waiting period, just seemed like more than I could bear. And I hadn't brought Paul along, because I really thought this was going to be very routine.

My poor doctor, who is ironically named Dr. Friend, was absolutely wonderful. Patient, compassionate and understanding. Kaiser seems to have more than their share of these docs, and I think it's the culture there. One of the reasons I like it so much.

Anyway, I usually like to be the ideal patient. Not this time. Not only did I break down in tears, but I screamed like a banshee when she did the biopsy. I'll spare everyone the gory details, but let's just say this was a spectacularly painful procedure, since I hadn't prepared by taking pain meds and valium like I did a year ago (yes, I've had one done before).

So much for being a rock star.

But then the afternoon came, and yet another doctor appointment. This one with the dermatologist, because while everyone's been staring at my nose and face ad nauseam the past three months, I was overdue to have the rest of my body checked for suspicious growths. After my morning, this was a much scarier proposition.

I'm really not worried about having uterine cancer. My lady parts have always marched to the beat of their own drummer and I'm used to that.

But my skin had already betrayed me. I'm never sure what could be lurking there. It's going to be the fear I live with the rest of my life.

But happily, I got the all clear! What a relief! A big enough relief to make up for the crappy morning. A big enough relief to make me want to head to Yogurtland with my Aitch for a treat on a hot afternoon.

And as I checked out, Dr. Goldstein told the nurse to put

me on the MELF list. I did a double take. Say what? Did he just call me a MILF? Nope, I'm a MELF: Melanoma Follow-up patient, meaning I get priority for appointments. A small, but meaningful perk for my troubled summer.

But it gave me a good hearty laugh.

So, as Pink says:

> *"I got a brand–new attitude*
> *and I'm gonna wear it tonight.*
> *I'm gonna get in trouble,*
> *I'm gonna start a fight.*
> *Na na na na na na*
> *I'M GONNA START A FIGHT!"*

Fuck you, cancer!

Make New Friends, But Keep the Old

September 2, 2011, 11:11 p.m.

Let's start with the good news. As I believed, hoped and expected, my endometrial biopsy was negative. Yay! As much as I "wasn't worried," I had a good little crying jag when I read my doctor's email. I always cry at good news.

Dr. Friend, by the way, is worth mentioning again. She took the time to send me this email at 8:30 p.m. on the Friday night of a three-day weekend! She had hoped – but wasn't sure – she'd get results by today and promised to let me know ASAP when she did. She obviously did not want me to have to wait through the weekend. God bless you for that, Dr. Friend.

Speaking of friends, tomorrow I get to see my dear old friend, Ilene, who is in town from Minnesota for a wedding. I've known Ilene since kindergarten. She was my first real friend that I actually chose to be pals with (i.e., that was not the offspring of one of my mother's friends).

Together we made clothes for our troll dolls out of felt squares, fought over who would get Ken as their boyfriend in the Barbie Board Game, fantasized that we were married to the Beatles (I was a brat and insisted Paul was mine), and played spy games in the back of my dad's station wagon as we drove to the Dairy Queen on hot summer nights (anyone with an "X" on their license plate was a bad guy!)

I've only seen Ilene a handful of times as adults, but there is always something so warm and welcoming about coming together with her. Besides her innately sweet nature – and her very accommodating husband, Jay – I believe that there is a certain comfort in seeing someone who knew you from those very first days of school, assuming it wasn't someone who beat you up, of course!

Those are the friends who know you in a very specific – and very innocent – way that few others do.

Shortly after my surgery, Ilene sent me an amazing package of photos from our childhood that she had taken the time and trouble to have reprinted in large postcard size.

It was such a spot-on perfect antidote for facing a life-altering disease. And that was a gift that few other people in my life could have given me. She even took one particularly sweet photo of me at about eight years old in my favorite winter coat and put it in a frame, ready to stand right there in my living room and remind me daily of who I once was, and who I still am, and who I will always be – that slightly mischievous, kind of kooky little girl with the big smile.

I still look at that picture every single day. I'm so glad that tomorrow I will get to thank her in person!

Planning a visit with Ilene again reminds me of the old Girl Scout song (yes, we were in Girl Scouts together), "Make new friends, but keep the old. One is silver and the other is gold."

That memory started me thinking about this silver vs. gold thing. I always thought of my "old" friends as those I knew in school or as a kid or teenager. But there are women – and men – I've met as an adult who are absolutely "old" friends, and it suddenly dawned on me, once you pass the age of 50, even your newer friends are old friends!

Only someone I'd met in the last few years would I consider a "new" friend. And let's face it, you just don't meet that many new people after a certain point in your life. Not that it doesn't ever happen, but certainly the opportunities to create close friendships dwindle as we get older.

But I guess here's one of those weird silver lining things about this whole cancer mess. There are a few people who, through this very site, have become "friends" of a sort.

People I had not met before. They have history with Paul, and I've heard of them in stories about Paul's life BBC – Before Barbara Caplan.

They are the very definition of "new" friends. I don't know whom if any, of the people I've come to know through their kind messages on my guestbook will actually become "regulars" in the TV show of my life. But the point is, I plan to be around for a long enough time for those who do stick around to eventually become "old" friends.

And frankly, I've learned that it doesn't really matter at this point in life whether friends are new or old – to me, they are all gold!

Stuck in the Moment, and I Can't Get Out of It

September 5, 2011, 8:56 p.m.

Sorry to sound like a broken record – even if the record is U2 – but I'm at complete odds right now. I feel uncomfortable in my own skin for some reason, with free– floating anxiety about nothing in particular that I can pinpoint. I had nightmares last night and woke up feeling like crap.

Here's the paradox:

I had a wonderful weekend, spent an amazing afternoon Saturday with the aforementioned Ilene and her husband, Jay. It was so great to see them both – truly a pleasure. We had a great time.

Followed-up with a relaxing afternoon Sunday with our friends, Steve and Kathrin. I didn't have to lift a finger. All I had to do was enjoy the company of people who I like to be with, and eat good food which I did not have to prepare.

What's not to feel good about? And yet ...

I'm exhausted.

And I'm frustrated with being exhausted.

And anxious about being exhausted.

And sick to death of being exhausted.

And I know what everyone keeps telling me – my husband, my doctor, my friends – I've heard it all until I want to scream! You've been through a trauma, you've had major surgery, your body is healing, you've taken an emotional hit ... and on and on and on.

Intellectually, I know all of that and know that it's right. But I'm just stuck in this place and I can't get out of it.

I'm sick of being stared at. I'm sick of my fake nose. I'm sick of waiting for the next thing to happen. Most of all, I'm sick of being tired and I'm sick of myself!

My dear friend, Vicky, who has gone through every single joy and trauma with me since the 6th grade and probably knows me better than any human being on the planet, with the exception of Paul and my sister, said something very revealing to me today. Vicky has provided me with some of the most amazing and valuable insights into myself over the 50-plus years of our friendship, and today was another one of those lessons. Here's what she deduced when I told her how I was feeling:

"You," she said, "are an extrovert. Extroverts get a lot of their energy from being around other people and socializing. But right now, you aren't really able to do that in the way you usually do. And worse, being around other people now actually drains you, so your whole world is kind of upside down."

And click! The light bulb went on. So brilliant, so true. Of course, it doesn't hurt that she's a mental health professional.

No wonder I'm so frustrated. You've heard of Mercury being in retrograde? Well, I feel like I'm Barbara in Retrograde! Everything's backwards and wrong.

But in an effort to gain some perspective and put myself back in a place of gratitude, I did have one realization on my own today. I was thinking about how sick I am of being stared at everywhere I go, and how I keep telling my friends, once I get my prosthetic, things will go back to normal, the new normal, of course.

Well, what about the people who don't ever get to "go back to normal?" What about the people with horrifically scarred faces? What about people who have an abnormal limb? Remember beautiful Bree Walker, the L.A. newscaster with the weird webbed hand that you just couldn't help but stare at while she was doing the news?

My hats are off to those people. I don't know how they do it. Sometimes I really don't care that strangers are staring, but there are other times when I wish like crazy that I didn't attract any attention in public at all.

My gratitude is for this: My freak-show will be over in a few months – I hope. Even if you can tell I'm wearing a prosthesis, it shouldn't be obvious to everyone until they look closely, and many people will never even figure it out.

If I can just find the patience to get there.

Good thing I married someone who has more patience than I do. I'm not sure where he's getting it from, but he seems to have found a well of it deep enough for the both of us.

This is sort of a non sequitur, but he's so patient. How patient is he? He's so patient that he stood at a kiosk with me in Century City for half an hour while I debated about which of two hats to buy. He even gave me his opinion and pointed out that one of the hats was marked SPF 50 (which I hadn't noticed and was the entire purpose for purchasing a hat in the first place!) And he didn't get irritated or antsy or pouty or annoyed. Or if he did, he hid it well, which is just as good.

Yup, that's my Aitchy. Best husband ever. And that's my other gratitude for the day.

I may get stuck in the moment again and again as I go through this process, but I will keep doing everything I can to be mindful of the multitude of blessings in my life. It's the only way I know to get out of it.

Flow It, Show It, Long as God Can Grow It, My Hair

September 6, 2011, 3 p.m.

Once upon a time, a little girl named Bunny had a lovely head of very fine, long golden hair. It looked very pretty but was very hard for Mama Muriel to get a comb through. Lots of hair snarls equal lots of tears.

So off they went to the beauty shop, where little Bunny's golden locks were shorn into a pixie. Oh, then the tears really flowed! Little Bunny had loved her hair. It made her feel like a beautiful princess. And now it was all gone.

But hair grows back. And when it did, Mama Muriel knew she would never get little Bunny to go to the beauty shop again. So, she hatched a scheme with sister DeeDee to "play" beauty shop at home. DeeDee, always good with hair and a scissors, was happy enough to do a hatchet job before little Bunny even knew what was happening.

Again with the tears. But this time came a vow. "When I'm big, I'm going to grow my hair out as long as I want and never cut it again!"

Of course, she got older, though she never actually got "big." And that's exactly what she did. As little Bunny grew into a teenager, not only did her hair grow, but her nose did too.

It grew until little Bunny became quite self-conscious about it. Thank heavens for the crowning glory of hair, which helped overshadow the fact that Bunny's nose had grown too big for her face.

Bunny's hair continued to grow until it was all the way

down to her tush. Everyone admired it. "You have such beautiful hair," people would say, and Bunny would beam with pride.

Fast forward 20 years. Bunny is now Barbara and finally, finally, decides it's time for a new nose. The plastic surgeon does a fine job and Barbara is happy, for the first time ever, really, with her new face.

Suddenly, she is free. And before long, she visits her hair stylist, holds her hair in her hand and says, "Take it all off!"

Friends are shocked, but love the cute new "bob" she sports, and for the next 15 years, she changes her hair regularly – a short little do just below the ears, shoulder-length, an angled bob, a layered bob – a whole world of hairstyles are open, and Barbara is intent on trying them all.

One day though, at the end of last summer, she misses having the flow of hair, and decides, quite out of the blue, to grow it long again. Many people consider long hair age "inappropriate" after 50, but she doesn't care. And grow her hair she does.

However, over a certain age, women's hair starts to change. It gets dry and brittle, or wiry. Sometimes it thins out drastically. But not Barbara's hair. She's blessed to discover that she can still grow healthy, flowing waves. Now, with her "revised" nose and her long hair, she again likes what she sees in the mirror.

And just when she's feeling all pretty even with crow's feet and a wrinkly neck, the evil cancer comes and steals her nose away.

Looking in the mirror is a whole new experience, but there is one saving grace. One thing that makes it not so bad. One thing that lets her still feel good – and that one thing is her head of healthy, flowing waves that gently drape past her shoulders and down her back.

What angel had whispered in her ear last fall? What twist of fate made her decide? What circumstance had led to her to do something that would become her safety net?

She could not have known last fall when she made the decision to grow her hair, that she would need it as her safe haven. She could not have guessed what was around the corner.

And long hair does not appear overnight. It takes months and months to reach below shoulders and beyond.

But Barbara knows with certainty that if she had not done so, if she now had a short stylish little "do" instead of long, flowing locks, she would feel naked to the world at a time when she could ill afford to be so exposed. Instead, she has all her beautiful hair to hide behind.

And now she stands before the mirror every day, combs her layered waves, and says "thank you," to God, the fates, and the universe that somehow led her to make the choice when she did.

> *"Give me a head with hair, long beautiful hair.*
> *Shining, gleaming, streaming, flaxen, waxen.*
> *Give me down to there, shoulder length or longer*
> *Here baby, there momma,*
> *everywhere daddy, daddy ...*
> *HAIR!"*

You'll Never Walk Alone

September 10, 2011, 12:45 p.m.

Of all the Broadway and movie musicals I have loved, Carousel was never a favorite. And this particular song, which moved so many to tears, always seemed just a tad too melodramatic for my personal tastes. Maybe in my previous life as an agnostic, it felt too religious and righteous, since it's supposed to be about God always walking beside us (at least that was my interpretation).

Well, I was thinking about this past week and this song suddenly popped into my head, but with a different spin that gave me new respect for it.

For months now, I have been on quite the journey and as I've said before, one of the biggest reasons I've been able to walk this path, as opposed to stumble, crawl, drag my-self along it, is because of all the incredible support I've had from family, friends, bosses, and of course, none other than my amazing Aitch.

This web page is my daily crutch where I get to see and read and feel how many people are behind me, pushing me through this dark tunnel towards the light.

But this past week particularly has brought a plethora of support from friends and in rather unusual and subtle ways.

First, there was the terrific visit with Ilene and Jay, which you've all read about.

Then, I finally got to have a phone conversation with my friend, Kathy, who moved from L.A. to Denver some years ago, but we still stay in touch. Kathy is also a writer, and she and I used to hike in the mountains while having terrific discussions on politics, morality and spirituality. I do so miss those walks and talks!

In our first real conversation since my surgery, the subject of "why" came up — actually, why things happen to people, and whether people "create" their reality, or if shit just happens randomly. It was a wonderful, thought-provoking talk that I will continue to ponder for some time to come. Though my feeling on this is generally: The "why" doesn't really matter at this point. It's how I choose to respond to what has happened that is really the crux of the matter.

Kathy does not really agree with me on this, and she is one person with whom I can disagree and yet not fight. The very fact of having a friend like Kathy with whom I can debate such points is a form of pushing me along my path, especially since our debates come from a place of love and friendship.

Then I had an exhausting, but "worth every minute of it" visit with long-lost friend Naomi and her husband, Marc. They were visiting from Canada, passing through L.A. on the beginning of a road adventure through many of the western national parks.

It has been nearly 40 years since Naomi and I last saw each other. Long story, but growing pains and many moves cut our connection, which I feared was lost forever until happily, the magic of the internet brought us back together ten years ago. And in our first conversation after all that time, we were just as bonded as we had been so long ago.

The world is certainly a "global village" now with people constantly communicating via phone and internet, but there is nothing like standing face-to-face with a person you love and spending actual time together over a good meal. The renewed memories, the joy of where our lives had gone — we both happen to be living very happy lives and are married to wonderful men — and our ability to still be as connected today as we were so long ago was a gift that really lifted me out of the depression I had been fighting recently. The bonus was having even more thought-provoking conversations with Naomi and Marc – and Paul, of course – about the nature of life and what happens to us.

But the most unexpected, and most bizarre form of friendly support came from someone local – I'll call her "Sally" because I don't have any friends named Sally and I'd like to protect her privacy.

Sally contacted me with a dilemma. She needed to gain clarity, wanted to hear a "voice of reason" about a situation she'd been dealing with. I got an email: "I need to talk."

I got this email in the middle of my visit with Naomi, and frankly thought there was no possible way I would have the energy to help someone else dissect a problem, and I didn't even know what the issue was. But I did call after Naomi left, thinking perhaps it was something quickly dispensed with.

It wasn't. Sally and I were on the phone for a good hour. But several wonderful things came out of it.

First, it was so nice to be needed by somebody else, rather my being the needy one. It was great to feel helpful for a change.

But much more importantly, by the time I hung up, I had a great realization. Sally's problem related to being stuck in a place she didn't want to be –the subject matter (relationship, work, living situation) wasn't even important – she's not happy in the place she's in, but isn't sure where she is going – and that's the amazing part!

SO AM I!!!!

I realized it's not just me and my cancer mess that feels this way: in limbo, stuck, not moving forward, etc. This is a fact of life for many people in many aspects.

I am not alone!

I hate the old adage that "misery loves company."
I would never, ever feel good about any of my friends
suffering. But having others in a similar situation certainly
does make you feel less isolated.

If you are lucky enough to have true and wonderful
friends, you can walk through a storm, lift your head up
high, and not be afraid of the dark, because there's a whole
slew of people walking through their own storms, but they
can still be right there beside you.

P.S. I feel a bit odd writing about myself on this weekend, when all the world's eyes are turned to New York on
this meaningful anniversary. I just want to take a moment
to remember those lost on 9/11 and to honor the brave
men, women and dogs who worked so long and hard in
the aftermath on such dangerous terrain. Many of them
are now fighting their own health battles because of their
heroism. Remembering you all on this somber weekend
with love and gratitude.

Like a Virgin (Hey!)

September 12, 2011, 10:59 p.m.

No, this is not an entry about a date night. "Virgin" in this context refers to doing something for the first time, and this past week has been a week of firsts.

In my pre-melanoma life, I used to do what I call "the working girl's spa day." I'd head for Century City, hit the Origins counter at Macys for a free facial, then follow it up with a stop at the massage chairs and let the Chinese guys work me over for 20 minutes. Voila'! For $15, I was a new gal.

But this summer, while dealing with the greatest stress of my life, I was robbed of my ability to do that. There was no way I could show up at the Origins counter for a facial with this giant thing on my face, and absolutely no way I could put my face with its delicate skin graft in the donut hole of a massage chair.

While the latter is still true until my face heals, the former was really more about my state of my mind than about logistics. As my surgical site shrinks, I've been able to reduce the size of my TFN, allowing more of my actual cheeks to show. And last Friday, I finally got over myself, marched on over to the Origins counter and said, "Hey, you can't get this wet (pointing to my TFN), but can you still do a facial?"

"Of course! I'd be happy to do it for you," was the response. And there, in the middle of Macy's, I settled back into their chair and let someone work on my face.

This doesn't sound like that big of a deal, but oh, let me tell you, it was a very big deal indeed. I went by myself (no hubby buffer), and I trusted a stranger – both with my face and with my psyche – and came away the better for it. It is, without question, one of the most normal things I have done in two months, and it felt damn good!

Today I jumped another hurdle and took an appointment with a new closet client – not a repeat, not a referral – an absolute stranger. I was nervous, to say the least, but I did it! I knocked on the door and said hello to someone who had no preparation for the weird fake nose that greeted them.

The lady was very nice, but the job was a complete bust. She wanted something tiny that we don't even do, but I was actually fine with that. It was a baby step. I got to have the experience without the pressure to design and sell all at the same time. My toe was dipped into the water and I didn't drown.

The next one will be easier.

Finally, this afternoon I did one more thing in the name of beauty. We have a huge family wedding this weekend. Very chichi, very formal (evening gowns required), and the one thing I've learned these past two months is that the best way to compensate for the mess in the middle of my face is to make the rest of me as gorgeous as possible.

To that end, I Grouponed my way to Billion Dollar Brows today and had my eyebrows shaped. Once again, I marched in and turned myself over to a stranger who had to work very closely around the top of my TFN. I did tell her the story and she was lovely about it and did a wonderful job. Now, at the wedding not only will I be decked out with a bejeweled TFN (stick-on rhinestones, thanks to Joy Johnston), but my lovely new eyebrows will enhance the overall effect.

(Sidebar: Did I really just turn Groupon into a verb? If all of my old English teachers aren't dead yet, this would surely kill them!)

And tomorrow will bring another first – a company meeting for all designers. My first face-to-face encounter with my colleagues, most of whom have no idea why I completely disappeared off the "Diamond List," the weekly email naming designers with top sales, where my name could often be found. They probably all think I quit since there isn't a lot of communication between us except at meetings, so fielding their questions may be a bit daunting.

It's a lot, I admit, and I'm feeling it keenly in the energy department. But as tired as I am, I am in a better place emotionally these last few days. Despite the toll it takes on me to do these "firsts," it represents something important to keeping me sane: Forward Movement.

And more is coming. Wednesday I'm seeing my surgeon and here's the first on my list of questions for him: Am I healed enough to put my face in the donut hole of a massage chair?!?!

If the answer is yes, it won't be long before I'm headed for Century City.

And if the doc says no, I'll just have to wait on that one. In the meantime, I've got bigger fish to fry. Tomorrow I'm just a week away from UCLA and meeting with prosthodontist! Woohoo! Now we're talking forward movement!

I'm so ready to get this party started: Let's scrap Madonna and crank up Lady Gaga!

> *"I'm on the edge of glory,*
> *and I'm hanging on a moment of truth."*

Extra, Extra ...
Read All About It

September 14, 2011, 9:47 p.m.

Very tired, so this'll be a quickie update.

Saw the doctor today. All good news. The Surgical site is healing very well. The little spot where the bone was showing now been mostly covered over by skin, so that's a big thing, as another procedure might have been required if it did not right itself on its own.

No follow-up again with him until November. He has officially turned me over to UCLA. It's now all in the hands of Dr. Kelly, the prosthodontist from Brainerd, Minnesota – nice to be in the hands of a fellow Viking!

And had The Good Dr. Kelly not informed me early on that he was a Minnesotan, I would surely have known it anyway from his repetition of the agreeable, "Yup, yup, sure, sure," uttered with an accent heard only in the upper Midwest.

Ah, he's my homey. Can't wait to see him. Cross your fingers, pray, sing, dance, whatever it is you do to bring good ju-ju when I meet with him.

I need a nap now so badly. But a nap this late is basically just going to bed early. Sleep tight, all.

P.S. Almost forgot the most important thing! I'm cleared to stick my face in the donut hole of a massage chair! Woohoo! Oh, Chinese guys at Century City, here I come!

The More I Change,
The More I Stay the Same

September 15, 2011, 8:27 p.m.

When I began this journey, I swore it wasn't going to change me. Then I realized, of course it's going to change me! I have a new reality that I have to adjust to. My life is permanently altered and there's no getting around that.

I have examined the subject of change in these journal pages on many occasions, and I'm still struggling with this issue.

I'm still me, I'm still the same Barbara. But I'm also changed. How can I be both changed and still the same?

Well, I may have finally come up with an answer. Here are some ways in which I am indeed both:

1.) How I've Changed: I'm never going to buy white underwear again. I love fun panties. I always have some pairs with flowers or paisley or stripes. I've always saved my "special" underwear for "special days." Well, no longer. Special underwear is for every day now. I know this idea is not original to me, but I'm stealing it from whoever wrote it first.

I once saw Rod Stewart wearing white pants and underneath, he wore red striped boxers that you could see plain as day! Hey, if Rod Stewart can do it ... (see my entry: "So What, I'm Still a Rock Star" from last week!)

How that proves I haven't changed: Life is supposed to be fun. I have always believed this. Obviously, I'm well aware that life is also hard work. But I've managed my entire life to always find some way to inject something fun into the midst of hard times. Wearing special panties shows I still have that core belief.

2.) How I've changed: I always wear a hat outside. I have a tiny head and could never find hats that fit, and never even thought hats looked good on me. It took years for me to feel comfortable just wearing a baseball cap. But now it's important that I shield my face from the sun.

How that proves I haven't changed: I love hats! I love hats so much that the heroine in my second novel, "Nothin' Left to Lose," had a thing for hats and always wore them. I gave her hats because, as stated above, I never felt I could get away with wearing them myself. Now, it doesn't matter how I think I look in them! (Once again, I refer you back to the "So What, I'm a Rock Star" line of thinking.)

3.) How I've changed: I seek the shade rather than the sun. I've always been something of a sun whore. I'm like a lazy cat. If there's a patch of sun, I want to be in it. Not anymore. I choose the shady side of the street now.

How that proves I haven't changed: I love myself; I love my life, I love my good health, and I will do whatever it takes to protect that. I have always been this way. That's why I quit smoking. That's why I go to Weight Watchers when I start to gain weight. That's why I gave up drugs. Hell, that's why I let them cut off my nose! I will not avoid the sun completely. But I will be extremely judicious about the ways and times I allow myself to be in it.

4.) How I've changed: I've learned to let people do things for me. I've never really needed anyone more than my two or three closest friends and my sister as my support system. But being diagnosed with cancer has brought everyone out of the woodwork. People have been amazing in their desire to want to do things for me, to help in some way – any way they can. And letting people do things for me has been something I've had to learn in a new way.

How that proves I haven't changed: I've always believed you have to let people do things for you – as a kindness to them; it allows them to feel useful. My father never used to let me buy him dinner; he always paid. It made me crazy and taught me how important it is to let others do things for you. But as I said, I've never been in such a needy position myself before, and therein lies the challenge I've worked to overcome.

I guess the point of all this is that the core of me is absolutely still the same. I have the same beliefs and philosophies about how to live my life and how to treat people and myself.

What changed are the accoutrements. The trappings of my own personal lifestyle and the way I manifest my philosophies are certainly new.

But I really shouldn't be all that surprised by the duality of my nature. I am, after all, a died-in-the-wool Gemini (see my August 21 entry). I have always been of two minds about most things.

About one thing I feel pretty certain. I've made my mind up over the past several days that I'm ready to take my life back. I can't wait any longer for the prosthetic to make everything all right.

I've babied myself, coddled myself, taken it easy, let other people do things for me, let Paul carry the lion's share of things around the house. I've needed to do that to heal.

But at some point, I have to – and want to – stop babying myself and fight my way through the obstacles holding me back: namely, fatigue and grief and insecurity.

My grief is not easy to dispense with and will continue for some time; perhaps it will always be with me. But I know from grieving my parents that life does not stop. At some point, you learn to put your grief in your back pocket and go on, letting yourself have it back only in private moments when it's appropriate.

My fatigue is a tougher battle to win, but I think it's time to push back against it a little more each day.

My confidence is clearly on the rise and grows with each new thing I take on. It's that very thing that will help me overcome the other two.

Saturday, I will sit at a wedding in a room with many strangers dressed to the nines. Five months ago, I would have welcomed the challenge of all those new people without batting an eye.

A month ago, I told Paul I didn't think I could do it, that he might have to go alone.

Now I know that not only can I go, but I will go and have a good time! Of course, I may fall asleep halfway through, but hey ...

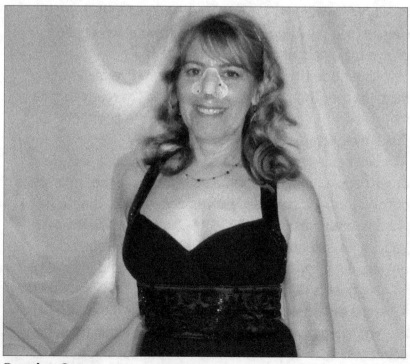

Dancing Queen

Dancing Queen

September 18, 2011, 10:31 p.m.

In our last episode, I was about to attend The Big Wedding. Well, it was last night, and all I can say is WOO HOO! I DID IT!

I, No-Nose Babette, attended our cousin, Chris's black-tie wedding at the Beverly Hills Hotel, joining Billy Crystal, Chris Rock, Larry David, Mayor Villaraigosa and Lu Parker, Kelly Lynch and some model whose face I know well but whose name I can't remember, all in their tuxes and gowns, as we dined in an elegant venue decked out with opulent rose and orchid floral arrangements, and best of all danced to a huge stellar band with back-up dancers!

And I did it all wearing my TFN bedazzled with sparkling rhinestones that drew compliments from a number of people!

Speaking of compliments: it was fascinating the number of people who told me I looked "stunning," "gorgeous," "beautiful," etc., repeatedly throughout the night. The amusing part of this was, as I commented to Paul on the way home, that had I not been wearing a fake bandaged nose, the strongest adjective I would have drawn might have been "lovely," "nice," maybe "pretty," or a compliment on my dress. It was my particular condition, I'm sure, that elevated the level of verbiage to hyperbole, but I'll take it!

I admit it. It did my spirits and confidence a world of good to hear it again and again. It was a wonderful and emotional evening for me for so many reasons.

First, I was surrounded by Paul's family, who are all incredibly kind and loving. Also, the bride and groom looked so happy, and to me, it's not a fun wedding unless the two people bringing everyone together are having a ball themselves – and they were!

Finally – and here's the frosting on the cake: I danced! And danced ... and danced ... and danced! I danced like a woman who didn't have a care in the world, like someone who hadn't almost lost her husband to sepsis in January; like someone who hadn't faced cancer and major surgery; like someone who hadn't recently lost a body part; like someone who wouldn't have to live with the specter of the melanoma returning.

For those who don't know me well, I've danced most of my life: ballet for years, followed by even more years of jazz. Though I no longer take class, a dancer is always a dancer, and the great joy of movement for me is the very manifestation of strength, power ... and good health.

In the middle of the evening, during a break from the dance floor, I was suddenly overcome with emotion, an amazing feeling of gratitude at my ability to dance again. I couldn't shed more than a few private tears without smearing my make-up, but for those few moments, I was overwhelmed with a sense of relief: relief that the worst is over, relief at the freedom I suddenly felt.

My feet and my body and my energy today all paid a very high price (we had to cancel dinner plans today because I'm toast). But it was so worth it.

Last night I truly felt like a dancing queen, young and sweet ... and only seventeen! (Well, plus forty.)

P.S. I wasn't the only Dancing Queen last night. The best visual of the night was Los Angeles Mayor Villaraigosa doing "The Bump," with Cousin Chris! Not everyone can say they've bumped asses with the Mayor!

Closer I Am to Fine

September 21, 2011, 4:51 p.m.

The long-awaited day has finally come and gone. Yes-terday I spent the morning with the UCLA prosthedontist, who declared me: HEALED!

Wa-hooooooo! Let the games begin. So, when do I get my new nose???

Of course, as the Indigo Girls say, *"there's more than one answer to this question pointing me in a crooked line..."*

As has been the case for this entire journey, there's good news and not–so–good news. The good news, as I said, is that I was sufficiently healed for them to begin the next step. They took a mold of my face so they can begin the process of creating the wax model to sculpt into my nose.

I met the artist who will be doing this, gave her pictures of how I used to look, etc., and we'll all be meeting again next week for the next step of sculpting. Very exciting!!!

The next piece of good news was that Dr. Kelly felt I might be a good candidate for clips or magnets! BIG YAY!!! As some of you may recall, I had my heart set on a magnetic "snap-on" nose. Yesterday, however, Dr. Kelly convinced me otherwise. Turns out clips are actually more secure and easier to maintain over the long-term. That's cool, as long as I don't have to deal with the daily mess and insecurity of a glue-on nose!

I also have to have several tests done to confirm that the bone structure in my head will allow a correct position-ing of the clips. Dr. Kelly seemed fairly optimistic, even said that my surgeon did an absolutely perfect job, but there's no guarantee until those tests are done sometime in the next few weeks.

Now the bad news: Because the clips are implanted into the bone, and because wearing the nose puts pressure on the clips, an adequate healing time absolutely must be allowed before the entire process can be completed. We're talking months.

My dream of being whole by the first of the year is beyond reach. If I'm lucky and qualify for the clips, I'm probably going to be wearing the TFN for another five or six months. This was a bitter pill to swallow, but the end result will be worth it. I would be very foolish not to go for the clips just because I was too impatient to get through the next six months.

As I lay back in Dr. Kelly's dentist-style chair, awaiting the mold to be taken, I had only a moment to consider feeling sorry for myself because of the lengthy process. I turned my head to look around and was startled to realize I could see into the next cubicle from my reclining position.

There, to my right, was a gentleman missing the entire left side of his face. I could see his lower teeth and tongue, but his upper teeth, upper palate, cheek, nose and eye were all gone. It looked as though a giant excavation had been performed on his head. My heart absolutely broke for him, and a sudden realization that six stupid months were so insignificant in the big scheme of things that I actually cried with gratitude that I'm so much better off than this poor guy next to me.

I saw them pour the mold into the missing half of his face and was amazed that they were somehow going to rebuild him. Un-frickin'-believable!

I ran into that man in the hallway afterward. He held a towel up to cover his missing face, so I could see only one eye peering out. I nodded at him and smiled slightly.

I wanted him to know I got it, I understood, that I am also a member of his club, albeit only a junior member comparatively speaking.

I didn't think of it at the time, but looking back, I wish I had put my arms around him and given him a hug. I don't even know his name, but the image of him has become like a kind of angel to me, my own personal reality check – my reminder of how unbelievably blessed I am and how narrowly I escaped such a mind-blowing condition.

I will still miss my nose (and oh, how I do). I will still get depressed. I will still feel bad when I need and want to because I have been through something awful.

But thanks to that stranger, I will never, ever forget how much worse it could have been.

There are still more questions to be answered. Will I pass the tests and qualify for implants? Will insurance cover it all? My conversation with member services today was very optimistic. I know that my state of mind and my mood will swing up and down depending on those answers.

I had hoped to have my nose by Thanksgiving. But I'm now hoping that I won't, because it will mean I'll be getting the implants. And at the very least, by Thanksgiving, all the questions will finally be answered and it will simply be a matter of time passing.

In the meantime, to finish the Indigo Girls quote:

> "The less I seek my source for some definitive,
> the closer I am to fine."

Long and Winding Road

September 26, 2011, 5:10 p.m.

Forgive me, readers, for I have sinned. It's been five days since my last journal entry ...

OK, I'm a nice Jewish girl who has never been to confession, but I've seen enough movies and writing this page does feel an awful lot like a kind of confession.

I truly miss doing a daily entry, but realized a few days ago that I've become too busy actually living life to write about it. That is, I believe, a very good thing.

Even though I'm trying to proceed with life as I used to know it, each day is still a challenge, still filled with many conflicting feelings. And each time I venture out the door, I encounter more inquisitive, concerned or just plain rude people. I'd like to say I'm used to it, no big deal, but it depends on the day and on my mood and on who's asking.

Yesterday, standing in line at a movie screening, a little old lady asked me in a conspiratorial whisper, "Who's your doctor?" I knew exactly what she meant – obviously wondering who did my plastic surgery as everyone in the whole world assumes.

I was tempted to say, "Which doctor? My oncologist or my prosthedontist?" But I didn't. I quietly told her I had cancer not a nose job.

When you tell people you have cancer, everyone's got a story. Their mother, their friend, their boss, their brother – someone they know has or has had cancer. Some days that makes me feel better; that person understands what I'm going through, and our shared experience means we can relate to each other on a higher level.

Other days, I want to say, "I don't want to hear your frickin' cancer story! This is my cancer and I'm the one who wakes up every morning without a nose!" Mostly I feel the former, but I am human and the urge for the latter response is there lurking on bad days.

I'm happy to say the bad days are less and less. I haven't had an 11 p.m. meltdown in a while.

I still have trouble getting through the day without a two-hour nap, but I'm trying to make them shorter and shorter.

I had another realization this weekend: It's been so long since I've had a regular face, that I've forgotten what it's like to look into a mirror and see something normal. This is normal to me now. By the time I finally get my prosthesis, it will be close to a year since I've had a real face. And I'm not even halfway through it yet.

I get weepy when I think of what it will be like to have a nose again. You've all learned I cry harder when I'm happy, but I'm having a very hard time imagining the sheer joy and elation I will feel when it actually happens.

I have another appointment with the prosthedontist at UCLA tomorrow. Every time we go, I get very excited like a child waiting to see when she'll get a pony for her birthday.

I have a new doctor at Kaiser now as well, the maxillo-facial surgeon who will be the one to tell me whether or not my bone structure will allow for workable implants (please, please, please say yes!). They can't get me in until a week from Friday. Then they will have to run more tests.

More waiting.

Endless waiting.

The light at the end of the tunnel is so far, far away, but it is there. And I'm hanging onto that with all my might.

I'm So Excited, And I Just Can't Hide It

September 27, 2011, 1:46 p.m.

This morning, the light at the end of the tunnel just got a whole lot brighter.

I saw my nose!

Granted it was made of wax and was bubblegum pink, but it was most definitely my nose.

It is absolutely incredible what doctors and artists are able to do. Dr. Kelly and the artist, Tomome and two interns who they were teaching, all stood over me as they placed the wax model on the surgical site and handed me a mirror.

I cried. You all knew I would, didn't you?

There, in the mirror, was ME!!! The "me" I haven't seen for so long. The "me" I said just yesterday that I had forgotten. But there was my face, a long-lost friend, staring back at me in the mirror.

Having the wax model on my face answered so many questions for me. After all, the TFN is uncomfortable and unwieldy – how could I know if the prosthetic would also be?

It's not!

Even though the model I had on was wax and not silicon, which will be used for the final prosthetic, it was much smaller than my TFN, more flexible and, thanks to the mold they took last week, fits just right and sits neatly in my surgical site.

I also spoke with Dr. Kelly about my chances of qualifying for the implants. He stressed that there is no guarantee but felt that they were pretty good. Unless I have some weird anomaly or malformation of the bones around my palate and upper teeth, I should be a good candidate. Only the CT scan will tell for sure.

It's hard not to count on this – I want it so badly. But I have learned to handle repeated disappointment these past few months and will reserve full elation until I receive final word.

The entire process that this whole thing entails is quite remarkable. Dr. Kelly is creating a new template of my nose that will provide a map of exactly where he would like the implants to go. I will take it with me to Dr. Tehrany's office – my Kaiser maxillofacial implant surgeon – so she will know exactly what she needs to do.

When I told Dr. Kelly it would be Dr. Tehrany handling the surgery, it was comforting to hear that he knew her, that she had, in fact, trained right there at UCLA, and that he felt she was very kind and caring, as well as being an excellent surgeon. Score!

It was a very good morning, indeed. I can wait now, however long it takes. Patience requires only a full under-standing of the desired and awaited outcome in order to be abundant. This morning, I have seen my future. And now I have something to hold onto until it arrives.

In the meantime, maybe I'll go play some Pointer Sisters and dance.

L'Shana Tovah Everybody

September 28, 2011, 8:22 p.m.

As the Jewish New Year begins, I just want to express my extreme gratitude to all of you who have kept me company through these past few months.

For those of you not schooled in Judaism, tonight begins the year 5772 (yup, we Jews have been around a long time), and although I'm not exactly the most devout Jew, I can think of no more important year for me to ask God, the Fates and the Universe to inscribe me in the "Book of Life" for the coming year.

Wishing everyone a happy, HEALTHY, prosperous and peaceful New Year. And if you are one who celebrates a different new year – then, Gung Hay Fat Choy (Chinese February), Feliz Ano Nuevo (Spanish January), or whatever will convey my very best wishes out there to you all for a happy "Let's Start Over" day. I used to know how to say it in Farsi, but I can't even begin to recall how to spit that one out here, so use your imagination.

L'shana tovah, everyone. Sending you all my love and good wishes.

It's Just Another Day, Doo-Doo-Doo-Du-Doo-Du

October 2, 2011, 8:56 p.m.

Once upon a time, people would ask, "What's new?" and I'd happily respond, "Not much, status quo, and I'm just fine with that."

This past year, first with Paul so sick and now the whole cancer thing, I haven't been able to say that in a long time.

People always think life should be exciting, and I agree we should all have some exciting moments, but frankly, I was always pretty happy with my low-drama situation.

Well, it struck me in the last few days, how close I am to getting back there. Yes, there's still the whole "implant or no implant" drama, but other than that, my life is pretty much back on track.

Just a few short months ago, I couldn't wash my face or my hair, I couldn't take a shower, it was hard to brush my teeth, my eyes were so wonky that my contact lenses didn't work, but I couldn't wear my glasses unless I taped them to my forehead.

Now, every day is pretty much business as usual. Showering in such a way that I don't get too much water in my sinus cavities has become second nature. I wash my face without caution or fear – even the skin graft, which is healed enough to be soaped and rinsed, and today, after a sneezing fit (a reaction to the blooming cactus flowers in our back yard), my nose-hole actually ran! Yup, for real! It was weird but comforting in an odd sort of way.

I am fine out in public now – no small thanks to my

successful attendance at the aforementioned black-tie wedding – and within a few weeks, I'll officially be back to work. I even managed to get through several days this week without a midday snooze. That's really progress!

But the true test of "back to normal" is my life with the animals.

First, our 16-year-old, three-legged Bailey had become completely weird the last few months, exhibiting extremely atypical behavior. The vet and blood work turned up nothing physical, and magically, in just the last two or three weeks, he has slowly resumed all his normal kitty behaviors.

As much as our animals are a comfort to us, and they are, (a recent study shows people with pets are better able to stave off depression), our pets also absorb and reflect back to us all the stress in their household.

It became crystal clear, as Bailey's return to normal mirrored my own, that it was my cancer and surgery that caused his odd behavior this summer. The vet confirmed this diagnosis, especially since we couldn't find anything physically wrong with him.

And finally, last weekend, I did something I haven't done in so many months: I attended a big Best Friends event, the Strut Your Mutt fundraiser for all the Los Angeles rescue groups.

Last year, I volunteered and spent quite a bit of time fielding pre-event phone calls and emails and working the "No More Homeless Pets" Information Booth at the actual event. I was slated to do the same this year, and very disappointed that I needed to bow out because of my surgery, but I knew I didn't have the energy to do a good job.

Returning to such an event, even as a visitor, gave me such a lift. I said when this journey began, that I'm not going to become "cancer girl," whose big mission in life is in the world of curing cancer – as noble a cause as that is. But I was determined that when I was well enough again, I would continue to follow my passion to help the animals. Spending time at Strut Your Mutt and seeing all my Best Friend "peeps," was another first step back into that part of my life.

BTW, thanks to all of you who donated to Strut Your Mutt through Paul's fundraising efforts. He collected the most amount of money for Best Friends L.A. team! It fell to him to carry the day for both Caplan-Bennetts.

It's amazing how much the return of routines, habits and passions can buoy one's spirits and push one forward on the road to being whole again. Of course, it won't all be final until I actually get my prosthesis next year, but believe me, having "just another day" is highly underrated.

Just ask Bailey, he'll tell you.

This Ain't No Party, This Ain't No Disco, This Ain't No Foolin' Around

October 5, 2011, 8:56 p.m.

Since I am out and about so much these days, a question keeps coming up: Why does it bother me so much that people think I "just had a nose job."

Virtually everyone who knows me remarks, when they see me for the first time, "Hey, no big deal. You just look like you had a nose job."

Many people even emphasize that since I'm in L.A., it's that much easier to get away with because there are so many women walking around who have had "work done."

I know friends and acquaintances mean to be comforting when they say this. Let me preface the remainder of this entry by saying:

If you are someone who has said this to me: NO WORRIES!!! I am not upset with you. You know what I've been through. But I am annoyed by strangers who automatically make this assumption about me. You would not believe how many strangers actually feel free to comment on my "nose job."

And I am is puzzled as to why this gets my panties in a twist!

I generally don't give a rat's patooti about what strangers think. But this – this one thing – it's like nails on a chalkboard to me.

But why? After all, I actually did have my nose done almost 20 years ago, and back then, I didn't care if people knew. Hey, it was no big deal at all, and I couldn't wait to

150

show off the finished product.

And maybe therein lies part of the answer.

There is a stark difference between the frivolity of a nose job where you are excited by the end result versus the trauma of cancer in which you are terrified by it.

I guess when people assume it's a nose job, it feels dismissive, like this is all a barrel of laughs that's going to have a fun outcome in which my new nose will be more attractive than the one I was born with.

Since my head is in a pretty good place these days, I would have thought that hearing the "nose job" thing would bother me less, but my negative reaction has not diminished, and I'm trying to understand it so that perhaps it will.

All I know is what I've said before on these very pages. I gave up my nose to save my life, and I'm permanently disfigured. The prosthesis will work wonders, but it will never be the same as having my own nose. Never.

And every time a stranger assumes I chose to have this thing on my face, I feel all the strength it's taken for me to get through this and live a public life is somehow discounted.

Maybe it's like this: When you work really hard to accomplish something difficult, the last thing you want is for everyone to think what you did was a piece of cake. You want credit for your hard work. Well, I guess that's how I feel.

This ain't no party, this ain't no nose job, and this sure as hell ain't no foolin' around – and I want the world to know I sucked it up, took it on the nose and came out swinging!

'Nuff said.

Whisper a Little Prayer
for Me, My Baby

October 6, 2011, 1:21 p.m.

Tomorrow I see maxillofacial surgeon Dr. Gabriella Tehrany, and although it's more than I can expect to come away from the consult with any kind of decision, at least it's a huge step forward in resolving the final remaining issue that still looms large:

Will I be able to get implants and a clip-on nose?

There has been no shortage of questions this summer with their own great import: Has the cancer metastasized? (No, thank God.) Did the skin graft take? (Yes, thank God.) Do I have to have radiation? (No, thank God.)

And now this. I've been so lucky, so blessed thus far. All the pieces have fallen into place all summer long. But I confess I am scared to death my luck will run out.

I understand this does not have "life or death" ramifications as the first question did, nor long-term healing and aesthetic questions as the second question did, nor even the long-term negative physical impact that the third question did, still ...

I have tried and tried not to have expectations about this, but the truth is, hard as I try, I want desperately to get those implants. I will have enormous difficulty containing my disappointment if the answer is no.

It's really almost silly. I'll still get a great nose. To the rest of the world, I'll still look pretty much the same whether it's glued on or clipped on. I don't know why I'm so fixated on this, but I am. I have been from the beginning, even though I originally thought the magnets were the way to go – same idea, no glue.

There are so many drawbacks to the glue – it's not as secure on the face, it requires a lot more maintenance and cleaning, and the glue can really irritate sensitive skin (which I have).

I guess it's that I believe I will feel a much greater sense of freedom and confidence with the clip-on – and as someone whose natural state is free and confident, that would represent a return to my true self; whereas I'm afraid with the glue I'll never really be me again in quite the same way.

Every step of the way, in recent weeks, I've been led to believe I'm likely to get the implants. Dr. Kelly thinks there's a pretty good chance barring something unforeseen showing up in the CT Scan.

I also just saw my dentist for a routine check-up and he took a look and said he didn't see any reason why it shouldn't work. He even went so far as to say if they couldn't put them above my upper teeth, they could probably put clips in the bones on the side. That upped my hopes another notch, though I take it with a grain of salt because he's my dentist, not my surgeon.

Tomorrow, the final leg of the journey begins. Saturday will be a very long day. It's Yom Kippur, a day of reflection, and the last thing I need right now is to spend a long day thinking about stuff. But I will rise to the challenge.

Sunday, I'm so grateful that my mind will be otherwise distracted since my sister will be arriving from Duluth. I'm excited for her visit, and we have some fun things planned (unless they get derailed by CT Scans and doctor visits, which could happen – and we're both OK with that).

I actually hope if I do get an answer on the implants, and the answer is "no," that I don't hear it while she's here.

I'd like to have her visit unmarred by bad news. On the other hand, if I could get good news while she's here – well that would just be so much sweeter!

So now, once again, I wait. Good news or bad?

Yom Kippur is not about praying to get something; it's about being sorry for any horrible crap you've done all year long (it's called the Day of Atonement for a reason). I'll certainly contemplate the things I'm sorry for: judging people, gossiping, being selfish and self-absorbed. But I wonder if I'll be able to restrict myself from sending out a prayer for implants.

After several weeks of being in such a good head space, feeling strong and resilient, I suddenly find myself feeling very vulnerable again. And I don't like it.

Watch this space.

I Can See Clearly Now

October 7, 2011, 6:26 p.m.

Well, it's a go!

Surgery to do implants is scheduled for October 31 – yup, Halloween. This time I will at least be a freak show on an appropriate day. Hey, if we get trick or treaters, I could answer the door and scare the pants off of them!

Our meeting with Dr. Tehrany was wonderful. Paul and I were wondering if our run of incredible doctors was going to hold out, and it did! She was a little blonde thing about my size, and after the towering presence of Drs. McNicoll and Kelly, it was a welcome relief to have someone on my eye level.

She was warm and patient and very encouraging. She said that one way or another, they would figure out a way to make implants work, hopefully in the easiest placement preferred by Dr. Kelly. But if for some bizarre reason the CT scan shows a problem with that area, there are other ways to deal with it.

Yes, Cousin Tom, DDS, you were so right, there are ways to do grafts and shift positions, and a bunch of other medical wonders to make it work!

Just from the examination she thought everything looked really good. It seems there's enough bone there, the skin graft seems to have taken really well. Everything is in place for it all to happen smoothly.

That's no guarantee, of course. She did warn that occasionally there are issues. Not every implant takes for a variety of reasons – infection, usually, but also problems can arise with the bone setting, or the skin graft losing

155

viability after being disturbed by the surgery.

But the odds are very much in my favor. She said there's about a 90 – 95 percent chance that all will be well. And if something does go awry, there are ways to fix it. It would simply prolong the process. But the end result will still be a clip-on nose.

WOO HOO!

And yes, I'm more than a little "ferklempt" at the good news. The road is no shorter than it was yesterday, but it is definitely clearer and more certain.

Being the night of Yom Kippur, I know that the beautiful Kol Nidre is being sung by thousands of Cantors in syna-gogues all around the world. But in my head, I hear only one song right now, repeating over and over:

"I can see clearly now the rain is gone.
I can see all obstacles in my way.
Gone are the dark clouds that had me down.
It's gonna be a bright, bright, bright sunshiny day

OK, I need to go cry some more now.

I've Got a Lot of Living to Do

October 16, 2011, 9:22 p.m.

OK, ten points for whoever can name the Broadway/ film musical from the '60's that spawned that song! Hint: Ann Margret's film debut. P.S. If the name Ann Margret is unknown to you, well, you're way too young!

Every day since I last wrote, I've wanted to sit down and do an entry, but first there was poker, followed by a visit from my Big Sis (yay!), followed by three days of some rather intense dealing with clients, and some random social activities including a friend's birthday party – making for a rather full week of living.

I can say with great pride that my life is absolutely, positively, back to normal (new normal, that is). As of November, I will be officially off disability and back to work, albeit not quite at full tilt for a while.

My social life has resumed pretty much as it once was. I've even stopped taking daily naps, though I still take them whenever I can get them. Part of my low energy, I've learned, is a mild case of anemia (who knew?), so I'm now taking iron supplements which should certainly enhance my ability to stay awake all day.

I'm happy to have been so occupied as it keeps my brain from working overtime on the journey still ahead. Two weeks from today is my next surgery. The last one took something away, this one will add something in, which is a good thing.

You all have heard me go on ad nauseam about the multitude of questions that keep popping up like a "Whack A Mole" game. As soon as I get one answered, three more appear. But at this point, it seems all the really big issues have been handled, and so now the devil is in the details.

I had a minor freak-out yesterday contemplating the possibility that my implants might not take because I'm on medication for osteopenia and there are some rare instances in which those meds prevent the implant from working.

I thought I was all good with not worrying about this surgery because I want it so badly, but let's just say the internet can be a dangerous thing. If you go looking for trouble there, you are sure to find it. Long story short, my perpetual voice of reason (Paul), and my retired dentist cousin, Tom (an early pioneer in dental implant work), managed to talk me down off the ledge. The reality is that only .003 percent of implants fail because of bisphosphonate medications. More importantly, the reality is that if Dr. Tehrany were really concerned, I'm sure she would have postponed the surgery until I had been off the meds for several months.

Of course, if I let myself, I can drum up a host of other things to worry about. But I can't control any of it, so I try not to go there. I've become an expert at pushing questions away that have no answers, with only an occasional freak-out.

Fear and worry are close cousins and learning to combat them both has forced me to draw on every ounce of strength I can muster. I'm on the down slope now, though, and that battle has gotten considerably easier.

I had several recent discussions with people about resiliency, and after my BFF, Vicky, called me the "Queen of Resilience," I started to wonder if there was, in fact, something from which I could not bounce back. If you had asked me six months ago how I would handle cancer and losing a body part, I would certainly not have believed I'd be "up and running" in my normal life in less than four months, and yet here I am, doing just that.

But as I pondered this question, I realized there is, in fact, one very big thing from which I would not bounce back, something so devastating that would crush me so severely, I'm not sure I could ever recover.

That would be losing my beloved Aitch.

All the strength, courage and resiliency I've mustered these past months have been exactly relative to how much I've been loved and supported by my husband.

Yes, the overwhelming support of family and friends was instrumental in my rapid recovery, and I thank you all for that.

But there is a way in which my Aitch has kept me aloft that no one else could – being with me 24/7 those first few weeks, in attendance at every single doctor appointment, consoling me at every single 11 p.m. meltdown, bolstering me through every single moment of doubt and fear. Rejoicing with me at every small and large victory along the way.

Once upon a time, when Paul and I got married, even though we were already middle-aged, he promised me at least 50 years. This is just a public acknowledgment that I fully intend to hold him to that!

In the meantime ...

*"There's music to play, places to go, people to see
Everything for you and me ...*

*Oh, life's a ball. if only you know it.
And it's all just waiting for you.*

*You're alive, So come on and show it!
We've got a lot of livin' to do."*

Anticipation,
It's Keeping Me Waiting

October 30, 2011, 4:42 p.m.

Wow! Two weeks since my last entry. So much has happened in that time, it feels a little overwhelming to address it all. So I'll stick to the pertinent stuff.

Tomorrow is the surgery to do the implants, which will provide the base for the mechanism to clip on my prosthesis – someday, a gazillion months from now when I actually have a prosthesis.

I had my pre-op with my doctor which, frankly, distressed me no end. After dealing with a full rhinectomy, I considered this surgery to be no big deal. Drill a couple of holes in the bone, set in the posts, voila'!

Turns out, not quite so simple.

There are a myriad of potential issues, in part because my teeth have very long roots, and also because they cannot place the posts in the optimum position, so they have to set them farther back, which creates potential interference by my one remaining turbinate (look it up) that I did not have to lose to the cancer.

Bottom line, they may have to move, trim or completely remove the turbinate. Also, the surgery may damage one or both roots of my front teeth necessitating one (or even two!) root canal(s), I will probably lose the feeling in my upper palate for some time until the nerve damage repairs itself – none of which I was prepared to hear, all of which left me feeling deflated and anxious.

Of course, NONE of these things may happen! And as my Aitch pointed out (as well as several friends), the doctors have to tell you all the worst-case scenarios to cover their asses. It only helped marginally to hear this, which brings me to my conclusion of the day.

It's all about expectations.

I was thinking about my surgery in July, which should certainly have been more terrifying, devastating, traumatic, _____ (insert dramatic adjective here). Hell, they were cutting off my nose, for God's sake!

Logic would dictate that I would've been much more stressed out about that surgery than this. Yet, here I am, worried, scared, and depressed that once again, things feel so out of control. Unlike my surgery in July, which I was expecting to be horrible, I was looking at this surgery as my savior. The thing that would give me what I want. The thing that would fix me. And it will hopefully still be all those things. I just wasn't expecting all the other stuff that might come with it.

I had been in such an incredibly good head space for so many weeks until I saw the doctor on Tuesday. After hearing all the possibilities, I suddenly felt just so tired of the whole thing. It's been months since I've had a normal face. It will be many more months until I do. I just want it all to be OVER!

But root canals, turbinectomies, numb palates – it all just seems like more stuff to get in the way of being done with the whole mess. So, there it is: my meltdown, the first one I've had in quite a while.

But there are two things that kept my week from being a disaster.

First, I got back in touch with my gratitude. I remembered all the things that could have gone south over the past few months but didn't. I didn't need radiation. The skin graft didn't fail. The cancer didn't metastasize. I just have to keep the faith. I'm hanging on by my fingernails.

The other bright spot to the week was my visit from BFF Vicky, all the way from Minnesota. When you've known someone for 51 years, there is an enormous comfort in being in their presence. Vicky knows every wonderful and rotten thing I've ever done, witnessed much of it in person, in fact. We've seen very little of each other in recent years but manage to keep our friendship thriving by telephone. She was an excellent distraction.

But now she's gone and reality is staring me in the face.

I will be very glad when tomorrow is over. There will still be questions, as always; I may not know whether I need a root canal for a days or weeks, but I'll have one more hurdle under my belt and be one step closer to the end ... I hope.

Cross your fingers, send good ju-ju, say your prayers, whatever your personal method of summoning good stuff is. You've all kept me aloft with your good wishes all these months. I need one more round (hopefully a final one) of support. Watch this space for the post-op report.

Hasta luego, amigos.

Surgery Report Via Texting With Paul

October 31, 2011, 2:27 p.m.
By DeeDee Widdes

I was hoping to never again have to do the reporting here, partly because I'm not the writer, my sister is. But mainly because that means she can't be reporting for herself.

Her surgery is over; she's currently in recovery. Paul said the doctor's report was good. As far as they can tell right now, surgery was successful, and they don't think any roots were hit. Only had to move the turbinate a little. They felt she should feel well enough to be up and about some tomorrow. She should be able to do the next report herself. One more hurdle behind her – yay! A little farther down the road to healed! What a relief.

Oy Vey

November 4, 2011, 8:36 p.m.

I just stared at my computer screen for ten minutes trying to think of something clever to put as a title, and that's all I could come up with ... which is, in itself, a statement about my condition.

You all know by now, surgery's done, went well, blah blah blah. But here I sit with a blood blister the size of a poker chip inside my upper lip. I look quite charming with my pouty swollen mouth, I must say. Angelina Jolie ain't got nothin' on me!

The two titanium screws shine brightly like I've just been bejeweled (so lovely), and I generally appear to have been hit by a semi-truck, although no other bruising yet, which is quite amazing, although the post-op instructions say bruising may appear after several days, so we'll see.

The worst part has been my throat. Something about the way they intubated me this time left me very raw and swollen and I have sores in my mouth – not sure from what. I'm having a lot of trouble talking, which might actually be a good thing for Paul.

Here's an appropriate place to insert my favorite line: "Other than that, Mrs. Lincoln, how was the play?"

The best part is that none of the things that I worried about seemed to have come to pass.

The doctor feels relatively positive she did not hit either root of my two front teeth, although root damage may not show up immediately, but so far, so good, and I'm feeling very positive about that.

My upper palate is not numb! I have full feeling there

and my sense of taste seems fine.

As for my turbinate, Dr. Tehrany was able to literally just push it a little farther over to one side so it's out of the way of where my prosthesis will go, i.e. she did not have to "trim" it, which would have been painful and yucky.

Yay on those three counts!

She also threw out something interesting that I am not going to bank on but will be eager to ask my prosthodontist. She seemed to think there was a good possibility that the bone will integrate with the implants in about six-to-eight weeks, as opposed to three or four months. Of course, she is not the final arbiter of the timing, Dr. Kelly is, but wouldn't that be an awesome surprise?

So now we're back in "wait and see" mode. After my post-op appointment with her on Monday, I'm going to try to get back into UCLA and have Dr. Kelly take a look to make sure everything is right for what he wants to do.

I Get Up, I Get Down, I Get Up, I Get Down

November 5, 2011, 8:36 p.m.

Well, if you've known me long enough, you knew I'd eventually get around to invoking YES lyrics. The album title, "Close to the Edge" seems fitting here as well.

It's been a hard week. Not like the worst week ever or anything. Let's not be melodramatic.

But I have not bounced back the way I hoped from this surgery. The idea that this was "no big deal" that led me astray with my expectations pre-op is apparently also responsible for my thinking I'd be feeling much better than I do post-op.

I had some unexpected bleeding the other night and spent an hour on the phone with Kaiser while they tracked down my surgeon. Turned out not to be too big of a deal because it eventually did stop on its own. But I confess, it freaked me out a bit.

In retrospect, I feel much more fragile than I'd expected to these past few days. One minute I'm fine because, after all, this surgery is a step forward to where I want to go. The next minute, I'm just sick and tired of being sick and tired. I guess it's a lot easier to knock me on my ass than I thought. And this has done just that. And I just realized why.

I've been using an awful lot of energy to keep myself in a good head space – and have done so quite successfully since I've been feeling physically well throughout October. But now that I'm not feeling physically well, there seems to be not a drop of extra energy to keep me emotionally afloat.

Every night before we go to sleep, I tell Paul that when I wake up I will have turned a corner and feel so much better: the sores in my mouth will be healed, my other various discomforts will have disappeared, but every morning I've been wrong.

The odds are with me, though. Sooner or later, I'll be right! I vote for tomorrow ...

In the meantime, I'm just getting through each day. Right now, having had anesthesia again, I'd really like to sleep all day every day, but that's not good for me. I'm really supposed to get up and move around a little bit. So, I think I'll go jump on the treadmill now and knock out a three-mile run. (Ha! And I have a bridge for sale in Brooklyn.)

Thanks, everyone, for your good thoughts and well-wishes. It really does help to know so many people are rooting for you.

I have to go ice my face now, but more and better stuff to come.

Back in the Saddle Again

November 7, 2011, 7:34 p.m.

The worst is over. OVER, I tell you, OVER!!!

At least that's what I'm choosing to believe at this point in time. I'm finally starting to feel like a human being again. All the various discomforts of the past week are fading.

I saw the doc today and she is very pleased with my implants and how they are healing. She had all good things to say about how the surgery went. All the things she warned me about did not seem to come to pass. I'm not entirely out of the woods yet and won't really be until we know for sure that the implants have completely set, but I'm far enough in the clear to feel confident that the hardest part is behind me.

There was originally talk that she might need to do a small additional skin graft to "cover" the implants, and then another surgery would be necessary to "uncover" them and put on the "healing caps." But Dr. Tehrany felt so good about how everything went that she went ahead and already put the healing caps on. So that's it! I'm DONE!

Of course, I'm seeing Dr. Kelly next week so he can have a look-see himself to determine if the implants are exactly what he needs. If it is, and I have every reason to believe it will be, since both docs have been working as a team on this, then it's really just about waiting for Dr. Kelly to feel the bone has set well enough to begin work on my final prosthesis.

We are still months away, but there is now nothing between here and there except check-ups: the dermatologist (who I have to see every three months forever), the melanoma specialist (who I have to see every six months forever), my surgeon (not sure how often on that one). But no more slicing, dicing or drilling! No more IV's. No more recovery rooms. No more pre-op, post-op or op-op. Woohoo!

As for being "back in the saddle," I am officially off disability now, back to work today, and already had to talk down an unreasonable client! LOL! Boy, it doesn't take long, does it? But no worries, I've got three wonderful repeat clients already needing me as well. So, I have an interesting week to look forward to.

In a couple of weeks, Paul and I will be taking our annual pre-Thanksgiving journey up the Central Coast to Moonstone Beach. This trip has always meant relaxation and renewal for both of us, but I think this year it will have special meaning.

Moonstone Beach is where I want my ashes to be scattered … someday. But as Aragorn said in "Lord Of The Rings: The Return of the King:" today is not that day! I mean, who wouldn't listen to the handsome Viggo Mortenson?

There was a brief moment in time this year, when we feared it was possible that day of scattering my ashes might be sooner than I ever might have expected. But that moment came and went, and now I have every reason to believe that I will have many live visits to Moonstone Beach ahead of me. I imagine it will truly feel like a fresh start on the rest of my life.

When we return from our time away and step into December, I am looking forward to a holiday season and a new year that are pretty much normal in most every way. After all, I'm only missing the final piece – my new nose. Of course, eventually I'll hit that milestone as well.

And I'm so ready.

On A Wonderful
Day Like Today

November 15, 2011, 6:02 p.m.

"I defy any cloud to appear in the sky,
Dare any rain drop to plop in my eye,
On a wonderful day like today!"

Yes, folks, it has been an amazing, wonderful day full of good news! Dr. Kelly was indeed delighted with my implants. There is nothing more to do but wait for the bone to set. I will be seeing him in mid-January to begin the lengthy process of creating my prosthesis.

He answered my numerous questions about the actual mechanics of the device I will be wearing, so I'm prepared now for inquiries any of you may have. (And anyone who wants to see pictures of the implants, let me know and I'll send them along, but you have to be able handle seeing my noseless face.)

The one, final little thing plaguing me after that good news, was that one of my teeth has been bothering me slightly (the bad one that's been hanging on by a thread for the past three years). Dr. Kelly took a look and didn't think anything horrible was happening, but suggested I see my dentist.

I was lucky enough to get in for an appointment this very afternoon because someone cancelled (it's been that good of a day!). After my dentist raised an eyebrow and speculated that the tooth may finally be "giving up the ghost" (which I couldn't even bear the thought of, more expense, another implant, more procedures), he did a further exam and decided that it was really just a simple matter of adjusting my bite!

I have a long history of bite issues and I wear one of those charming bite guards at night, so it should be no surprise that all the stuff that's been done to my face would throw my bite off a bit, and yet somehow, in the midst of everything else, it never dawned on me that it just might be that easy a fix. But it was!

So I'm not going to need extensive dental work, either!!! At least, I won't in the next few months. AND ... to really put the frosting on the cake, my dentist asked to see the implants and was absolutely blown away by how gorgeous the whole thing looks: the rhinectomy, the skin graft, the implants; he was positively raving about what an incredible team I must have had, and as he said himself, he is quite difficult to impress!

Nothing makes a gal feel better than having someone rave about the beauty of the big hole in her face! In fact, I'm thinkin', if there were such a thing as rhinectomy porn, I'd be the centerfold!

I am yearning to celebrate, and Paul and I were tempted to go out tonight and kick up our heels, but I have an enormous work project (another wonderful thing!) and I'm on a deadline since we're leaving town, so we'll save our celebrating for our upcoming trip away.

WAHOOOO!!!! I just don't have the words to tell you all how happy, how relieved, how ecstatic, how delighted, how thrilled I am.

Thank you, thank you, all of you, for riding along with me on this long, difficult journey. All of the good news, when I've had it, has been so much sweeter since I've had you all to share it with.

And of course, I can never end these posts without once again touting the three-legged blessings on which I've perched now for months: my incredible bosses, my incredible team of doctors, and yup ...

The ever–amazing, Super Husband, the Incredible Care-Taking Man, the King of Emotional Support, the Champion of Loving Acceptance ...

My One and Only Aitchy. I love and adore you and I don't care who knows it!

So sing along, everybody ...

> *"On a wonderful morning like this*
> *When the sun is big as a yellow balloon*
> *Even the sparrows are singing in tune*
> *On a wonderful morning like this."*

Life is Not About Waiting for the Storm to Pass

November 25, 2011, 10:19 p.m.

Thanksgiving week is my favorite week of the year. Paul and I always have our trip up the central coast, we see family at Thanksgiving, and we spend oodles of time hanging out together, doing whatever we want to do at any given moment, even if that means doing nothing at all.

I had enormously high hopes for the week. I had gotten the all clear from Dr. Tehrany, Dr. Kelly, and even my dentist. I had a wonderful client who gave me a big order as my final act of work before vacation – always a good way to go ...

And then the tables turned.

Right before leaving town – and too late on a Friday night to reach any doctor or dentist – I discovered my front tooth was turning gray and was starting to ache. I knew this was not a good sign, but I wasn't sure how bad it was either. I try, and I try, and I try not to worry about things I can't do anything about, but I really did not want to leave town with this hanging over my head.

Sometimes life doesn't offer you a choice. Either you go and decide you will enjoy yourself, or you let a nagging concern ruin a good time.

I decided to pop Tylenol like candy and make a conscious effort to achieve the first option. I am happy to say that I was mostly successful.

We did have a wonderful time at Moonstone Beach. We had some great wildlife sightings, which always just makes the trip for me. We had wonderful meals, we had gorgeous weather, I got clobbered in Scrabble ... and I got to just hang out with my Aitch.

One afternoon, we were in a little store in Cambria called Home Arts where they always have wonderful and unusual gift items. There I saw a pillow with a saying on it:

"Life is not about waiting for the storm to pass,
it's about learning to dance in the rain."

It hit home so hard that it brought tears to my eyes. I realized the biggest reason why I was so upset about my tooth was that I had decided all the bad stuff was over. The whole process that began with a biopsy in May was finished. All I had to do now was get my new nose. The proverbial storm had passed.

But that is not the case. Now I have one more thing to deal with. More questions, more time lost running to doctors and dentists, more expense, more pain, more recovery.

But reading this saying on the pillow made me realize this: hard times are part of life. There isn't really any point at which you can say they are over. Even if you, yourself are fine, someone close to you is always struggling or suffering or going through a rough patch. Which is why, especially why, it's so important to be grateful for the good stuff, to appreciate joyful moments, the peaceful moments – the times I like to call "low drama days," where we all kind of float along unscathed.

This week became a "dancing lesson" for me, and it was a damn good class. Of course, being the dancing fool I used to be in a very literal sense, I was once told by someone that I could dance to the sound of dishes breaking (he meant it as a compliment). And that is kind of what I did this week. I danced to the sound of dishes breaking.

On a final note, I had the amazing good fortune to get a free holiday consult with my favorite dentist in the world, my dear cousin, Tom, with whom we share Thanksgiving. He took a look at the tooth and gave me all the 411 on what might be going on. (And you all know me – knowledge is power.) He completely lifted my spirits by telling me that even if it's the worst case scenario (I need a root canal), it's the easiest tooth with the shortest appointment and the lowest cost – and you don't need a crown, they have another way to remove the gray. Thank you, Tom! It just simply is not that big of a deal.

Of course, I will really relax after I see Dr. Tehrany on Tuesday and she tells me that everything with the implants is still OK, weird dying tooth notwithstanding. But I have every reason to believe it will be a confirmation that all is well.

In the meantime, I have two more days of bliss, and I have the best dancing partner on the planet, so I'll just keep dancing.

Which One's Not Like the Others

November 30, 2011, 8:36 p.m.

The Panama Canal. The Erie Canal. The Root Canal.

Well, it's official. After weigh-ins from my cousin, my surgeon, my dentist, my Aitch, both cats and that weird voice in my head that speaks whenever my tooth aches. I'm having a root canal at the end of next week.

Wish it could be even sooner, because right now, no matter what time it really is – is it still just 2:30? (Get it? Tooth-hurty? LOL. OK, my bizarre sense of humor has run amuck!)

So, why the root canal? Well, according to my dentist, he believes the tooth is dying from trauma it sustained during my original surgery back in July (the rhinectomy). Many times he has seen patients after surgery with broken, cracked or dying front teeth from the intubation process. Apparently, intubating can require some wrestling and the front teeth may get knocked in the process. And a dying tooth takes some months to show up, hence, his belief that it was the first intubation that caused it (as my brilliant Cousin Tom also surmised).

The good news? Yes, there is always good news ... my implants are just great. No signs of infection or rejection. Dr. Tehrany was pleased that they look so good, so all the important stuff is cool.

And I do have dental insurance. Of course, it's one of those where they pay a percentage of the "scheduled" fee: i.e., your root canal costs $1,250 in L.A., but their fee schedule says it only costs $750 because that's all they might charge in Podunk, Iowa. Still and all, I'm grateful to have anything that will help defray the cost.

In the meantime, the rest of life is just fine and dandy. I had a terrific first month back at work. Surpassed all the goals set for me by my boss. Earned a nice bonus. It feels wonderful to be a contributing member of the family and society again, instead of a noseless bump on a log.

We are even adopting a new family member this Friday. We've been wanting to do it for months because Bailey is too old to play now, and William really wants someone to chase and tumble with. But dealing with all the cancer stuff has just made it impossible to even contemplate, until now. We are adopting a beautiful black cat whose final name has not yet been determined. We're keeping our fingers crossed that the boys will accept her, after a proper introduction, of course.

She was pulled from the shelter by a rescue group with her six kittens, who were all adopted. She has been in a foster home for over a year. At two and a half, she's old enough to be past the manic kitten energy, but still lively enough to give Big William a run for his money. Somehow, it seems fitting to bring a fresh dynamic into the house now, shake things up a bit.

I know a new cat is not exactly on topic for a website to share news about my cancer, but in way it is. Bringing this girl home is another step in the return to normal life.

As for my root canal: eh, it's really not a big deal. A new animal friend? That's a big deal.

And here we are already at December. Going on six months without a whole face. But the months are flying by and we're heading for that wonderful new nose, then straight on 'til morning.

It's Hard to Dance with the Devil on Your Back, So Shake Him Off

December 5, 2011, 7:32 p.m.

Thank you, Florence, and thanks to The Machine as well, for providing the soundtrack to my life these past few weeks. And thanks to my Aitch for being such a hip old man and playing the CD nonstop in the car.

It is, indeed, hard to dance with the devil on your back, and I've had a rather tenacious devil on mine.

Warning: Whining ahead ...

I'm so sick of the word "challenging," but there is no better word to describe what's been happening. I haven't written in so long because, well, I was sick as a dog, and frankly, I've felt beaten down and just had no desire or energy to be communicative.

When I have nothing positive to say, it's hard for me to say anything at all.

To catch everybody up, after my last entry, I developed a horrible sinus infection. After four days of fever, I realized it was not going away on its own, got myself to the doctor and got me some fine antibiotics which knocked that old infection on its ass! Lord, drugs are amazing things.

In the meantime, I also had my root canal.

I am now, finally, at long last, without pain (for the first time in weeks), and without grotesque amounts of snot, and without any other debilitating physical circumstances. But still, the emotional lethargy lingers.

I said to Paul today that I think I must be somewhat depressed, because I just don't want to do anything. I just want to hide out and watch TV. We were pondering the whys and wherefores of my feelings and I guess I'm just completely out of any reserves to bounce back yet again. Sure, a sinus infection and a root canal are really not that big of a deal. They are run of the mill, everyday maladies that all people deal with.

But for me, they have much bigger implications. And it's all about the implants and keeping them healthy and strong while they become one with my bone. With any kind of nasal infection, the question is one of keeping everything clean, which meant repeated removal of copious amounts of disgusting stuff from the big hole in my face. I should have bought stock in Q-tips; I've gone through so many applying disinfectant to the areas around the implants.

As for the root canal, well, again, it's all about the implants – the doctor's admonitions to be sure my endodontist doesn't overshoot the root and disrupt the titanium screws – the concern that any infection in the root could disrupt the healing and ultimate success of the screws. But I do have an excellent endodontist. He did a sterling job. He even got rid of the discoloration of my tooth with a bleach plug that worked perfectly, so my smile is bright once again, and the pain is gone. And I even saw on the x-ray that everything is safe and sound.

So, in the end, all's well. And I would say all's well that ends well, but it's just not how I'm feeling at the moment. I'm feeling that I wish things would just be well all along, not just end well.

It strikes me as sad that I no longer feel like everything's going to be fine once I just "get past this." I don't trust anymore that I will ever be "past" the bad stuff. It's like my quote last time about not waiting for the storm to pass, and when I wrote about that, I had plenty of emotional strength to acknowledge and accept that is life, but right now ... come on!

I'm ready for a bit of a break.

I'm also sick of being stared at, and I swear, if one more person tells me I'm an inspiration, I'm going to scream! I don't want to be an inspiration, I just want to be plain and boring. Paul says I can't help it, it's just who I am. And I guess I am happy if I'm inspiring someone to visit their dermatologist or put sunscreen on their kids. But yikes! Isn't it somebody else's turn to be inspiring?

There are people who have it worse, I know. But I feel very self-absorbed at the moment and can't quite bring myself to feel better just because others have it worse.

Tomorrow I see Dr. Tehrany. She will assure me that all is well and that the implants look great, and that I did a stellar job of keeping them clean (obsessive compulsive behavior can be a good thing sometimes). And on January 17, I will return to my prosthodontist to begin the lengthy process of creating my final nose. I can hardly wait.

I am SO fucking sick of wearing this plastic thing on my face (pardon my French). And poor Paul is sick of hearing me say how sick of it I am.

While I wait for January 17, I'd like to just change my name to Rip Van Winkle and take a really, really, really long nap.

But the new year will come, I will bounce back, because I always do, and then maybe Florence and the Machine will be right when they sing:

"The dog days are over, the dog days are gone.'

No Day But Today

December 20, 2011, 3:52 p.m.

I don't know how, I don't know why, but today, this song from "Rent" that I love so much popped into my head.

Perhaps it's the universe reminding me to be in the moment, to stop feeling badly about what's happened in the past and just ... LIVE!

My BFF, Vicky, has been studying "mindfulness" recently and has been sharing that knowledge with me. Remembering the lyrics to *No Day But Today"* seems like a pretty good definition of "mindfulness." And it's a way of thinking I can really get behind. This is just an excerpt:

> *"There is no future, there is no past*
> *Thank God this moment's not the last*
>
> *There's only us, there's only this*
> *Forget regret or life is yours to miss.*
> *No other road, no other way*
> *No day but today*
>
> *I can't control my destiny*
> *I trust my soul, my only goal is just to be ...*
>
> *There's only now, there's only here*
> *Give in to love or live in fear*
>
> *No other path, no other way*
> *No day but today."*

*** *** ***

For those of you who don't know "Rent," it's a musical about AIDS. I first heard this song in the 90's, not long after losing my beloved friend, Jeff, to that horrible disease. It made me remember and appreciate the time I did have with him. It made me cry then to hear a magnificent chorus of voices belting it out on stage at the Ahmanson, and to this day, it brings tears to my eyes every single time.

Life is so fragile, but so amazing. What we get of it we must appreciate. One line in the song I do take issue with: "I can't control my destiny." While there are many things beyond our control, we do have more power than we know. The power to love and create meaningful relationships in which there is mutual nurturing and support. The power to keep our minds and our hearts open. The power to resist violence. The power to take action when we have passionate beliefs.

These are all ways in which we do control our destiny. But still, in the final analysis, there is no day but today.

I won't apologize for my last whiny entry. It was an honest display of my emotions at the time, but as Emily Litella (Gilda Radner) used to say on Saturday Night Live 30 years ago: NEVER MIND!

I'm off the pity train and back on track and wanted to share that with you all.

The guestbook responses and private responses to my last entry are very much appreciated. It's enormously helpful to have people understand that even Pollyanna can forget how to play the Glad Game now and again.

And in truth, I am honored if others are inspired by me. I don't have children, and what better legacy can I leave to the world than to create a positive influence on people.

Back to my life-saving mantra: find the gratitude!

And I am grateful – so, so, so grateful for the many blessings in my life. A fever and pain can make one lose sight of that, but all the reason to work even harder at being conscious of the good stuff. I still have the best husband on the planet. I still have incredible bosses. I still have amazing friends and family. I still have the best doctors. None of that has changed, which just goes to show ya, it's all in where you put your focus.

And, of course, an interesting thing happened on Monday. A mere one day after I declared myself sick to death of being told I'm an inspiration, the amazing (and adorable) Dr. Tehrany sat down with me in the exam room, looked me in the eye and said, "I think you should consider motivational speaking about your experience. There are a lot of people you could help."

Don't ya just love how filled with irony the universe is?

"No day but today."

I Used to Love Roller-Coasters

December 5, 2011, 8:05 p.m.

But I'm ready to get off this one.

Our beloved Bailey, our 16-plus year-old cat who has been with me and Paul for all but a few weeks of our entire relationship has a mass in his belly. It's not good. If you've never loved an animal like a family member, please don't even think of reassuring me by reminding me that I've survived my own cancer.

Our goal is to keep him comfortable and happy for whatever time he has left. We don't know whether that's a month or a year. Awaiting discussion with our vet for more details.

I'm heartbroken beyond words, but I will have to dig hard and deep to find the strength to deal with this, because I know how hard it's going to be on Paul. I hope I have it in me.

All You Need is Love

December 28, 2011, 12:18 p.m.

John Lennon had so many things right. This past year has taught me that this song was one of them.

I was lying in bed in the middle of the night thinking about how driven by fear the human race is and where that comes from. I have clients that are so fearful about the silliest things. It seems odd to be so worried about making aesthetic choices about your closet, and yet they are. They will literally put off making a decision that functionally could make a huge improvement in their lives just because they don't know whether they want large crown molding or small crown molding.

Fear is such a horrible waste of time. Not that I am without fear myself, certainly. And of course, fear is part of our survival instinct that has kept the species going for so long. But we should certainly be mindful (there's that word again) about what we spend our time and energy fearing.

Right now, of course, I'm dealing with fears about Bailey – how will we know when his time has come, etc. But he's doing well on steroids, and I'm trying to focus on each day with him, not the future, which is out of my hands.

But in the middle of the night, my thoughts return (as they often do) to dealing with my own disfigurement and it made me realize that, although there are many things people fear, there are really two big ones that drive everything.

We fear death, as I said, part of the survival instinct. But I do not believe we go through our daily lives with that uppermost in our minds.

Much bigger, much more pervasive: we fear not being

loved. This, I believe, drives just about everything we do. Being alone and unloved is terrifying for most people. And by being alone, I mean being truly alone. I enjoy my own company and am just fine and dandy doing stuff by myself and being left to my own devices. But I can be comfortable being alone because I know that out there in the world, there are people who care about me.

So, I applied the question to being disfigured: why is it so frightening? It really doesn't matter a hill of beans whether or not I have nose, physiologically speaking. I think we fear being ugly because we fear being unlovable.

The bottom line is that I got through this whole ordeal mostly because I happen to have the extreme good fortune of sharing my life with someone who loves me in a way that I never had to have that particular fear. Gee, I only had to fear death, though I got over that pretty quickly with a clean CT scan and brain MRI.

I've said to many people over the past six months that it takes a special man to make a woman with a hole in her face feel beautiful, but my Aitch does ... every day.

And then I have the added bonus of my family and friends who love me. But I've noticed a funny thing about that.

I've never been one to say "I love you" easily. Oh, I tell Paul all the time, and I tell the cats constantly, but when it comes to people, not so much. It's never rolled easily off my tongue, even with my own sister, who I have great love and affection for.

I'm not sure why I've been stingy with the "I love you's." I guess I would have to revisit my therapist to figure that one out.

I think part of it is because "love" has always meant a very deep emotion for me, not just something that you bandy about lightly. It's the same reason I spend an hour picking out a simple greeting card. I won't send one that says something I don't truly mean.

But throughout all these months, I've had so many people tell me they love me, that I've come to reevaluate the meaning of the phrase. There are many different kinds and levels of loving someone. And it's time I broaden my definition.

Perhaps love is like the Richter scale of an earthquake. A 5.0 earthquake is not one measure more than a 4.0 – it's ten times more. And every person who expressed their love for me throughout these past months, whether it was a 3.0 or 10.0 love, added exponentially to the support that pulled me through the worst of times.

In a way you could say, all I needed was love ...

And I'm so blessed to have so many people offer theirs to me in such dark times. So here it is, folks – in case I haven't told you enough before ...

I LOVE YOU!

Lost ... and Found

December 31, 2011, 3:55 p.m.

This year seems like one of obvious losses, yet it has also been a year of interesting discoveries.

As my farewell to 2011, I share with you all my list of Things Lost, Things Found, and Things I Thought I Lost, But Then Found Again ...

Things I Have Lost

1.) My nose (duh!).

2.) My sense of immortality: mostly my own, but also Paul's, and also Bailey's.

3.) My ability to swim with my head underwater, though the right snorkel mask may fix that. I just haven't found one yet.

4.) My ability to have a full facial, though the Origins mini-facial helps. Still, the delight of having my face and nose fully massaged during a facial is gone forever.

5.) My ability to bake in the sun on the beach or during a hike without giving it a second thought. I have become a prisoner of sunblock.

Things I Have Found

1.) Great gratitude and respect for the world of medicine, and especially my doctors.

2.) Enormous appreciation for the compassion of my employer (Closets By Design).

3.) A bond with my Aitch even stronger than I imagined it could be.

4.) The knowledge that I can, indeed, be strong in the

face of life's challenges as I always hoped I would be if put to the test. I was never really sure I could hold my own against cancer or disfigurement; now I know.

5.) More loving and supportive friends than I ever guessed I had. Several people told me at the beginning of this journey that I would lose friends, that there are some people who just can't handle cancer. To my surprise and delight, none of my friends disappeared, and in fact, people appeared out of nowhere to buoy my spirits through the most difficult months.

6.) Sadly, a hypervigilance about every lump and bump that appears on my body. No little black spot is ever going to catch me off-guard again.

7.) My voice. Thanks to the Caring Bridge site, I've discovered that I enjoy being an essa-yist much more than a novelist. I kinda, sorta already knew that, but having this wonderful forum has proved the point.

Things I Thought I Lost, But Found Again

1.) My dignity. I think this is self–explanatory.

2.) My whistle! Some of you may remember my writing about having lost my whistle, but then, with great effort, was able to find the muscles to do it again, but just barely. Fast forward a few months: about two weeks I ago, I found myself just whistling a jaunty tune without even giving it a second thought! I was amazed and so happy. I really thought I'd never whistle again without great effort.

3.) The little indent between the cupid's bow of my lips. For months now, the space above my lips has been puffy and kind of weird looking, and I thought it was just one more permanent change that I would have to adapt to. But just the other day, I noticed the puffiness had abated ever so slightly so that the little indent is beginning to reappear above my lip. Paul reminded me that the doctor said it would probably be a year or so before all the swelling would go away and things would be settled into their final shape.

4.) The ability to be the me I've always been. Someone rather unself-conscious, someone able to walk into a room of strangers with confidence, someone who doesn't mind being the center of attention (but doesn't need to be), someone who smiles – a lot. In an early post, I pondered how all this would change me. I feared I would shrink instead of grow because it would be so easy to do that. While there have been a multitude of small changes in how I think and my daily routines, I know now that Barbara (Bunny) Caplan-Bennett is fully intact.

*** *** ***

So, there it is. When I sat down to write this list, I thought it would be more revelatory, but it's actually pretty much what I've been saying for months.

My journey is slowly drawing to a close. I go see Dr. Kelly at UCLA on January 17 to begin the process of creating my prosthesis, so I'm guessing that in less than three months, this story, and this post, will come to an end.

I don't know what 2012 has in store for me. It will probably bring the loss of my beloved Bailey and that will be hard to bear, but I don't expect any year to be completely devoid of difficult things.

It is hard to imagine that even with losing Bailey, it won't be better than this year has been. But whatever does come my way, 2011 has taught me that I will probably face it head on and live to tell the tale. Because at this point, really, there's only one loss from which I fear would not recover – and thankfully, my Aitch proved his own mettle when he successfully battled sepsis this year, so I would hope I won't have to face that for decades to come.

In the meanwhile, time marches on. We all march on, through whatever fire life throws our way, and in the brilliant words of R. Crumb: let's all "keep on truckin' ..."

Sending you all lots of love and wishes for a safe, happy and healthy New Year!

Long Time Comin'

January 16, 2012, 9:35 p.m.

> *"It's been a long time comin',*
> *It's been a long time gone.*
> *But you know, the darkest hour,*
> *Is always just before the dawn."*

I believe David Crosby meant this to be a political song, but it comes to mind often when I've been waiting patiently – or impatiently – for something to happen.

Tomorrow is my appointment with Dr. Kelly at UCLA to begin the process of creating my prosthetic nose.

If you read this as having been written in a calm voice, let me restate it:

TOMORROW IS MY APPOINTMENT WITH DR. KELLY AT UCLA TO BEGIN THE PROCESS OF CREATING MY PROSTHETIC NOSE!!!!!

OK, I think that more accurately conveys my emotional state about now.

I have been without a whole face for so many months, I have worn that @#$* plastic nose for so many months, I have been stared at on the street for so many months, I have lived an alternate reality for so many months.

And while I've thought often about when this day would come, I could not allow myself to go fully into the depths of what it means to me because it was still so far away. But these past 48 hours, I find my emotional state becoming more and more intense. I find myself wanting to cry all the time – in a good way, in a happy way, a cry of relief.

You know how when you're about to go on vacation,

work suddenly becomes unbearable – or, for a slightly more visceral example, when you have a slight urge to pee but get within sight of the bathroom you suddenly have to go so badly that you're not sure you'll make it?

Well, that's how I feel right now. Every day when I tape that plastic thing to make face, I grow more and more irritated at the discomfort and inconvenience. Every day when people on the street do a double take as they pass me, my desire to look "normal" grows stronger.

Tomorrow the process begins. It may take six-to-eight weeks, maybe even ten if things don't go smoothly, but the end of this horrible journey is in sight.

Kind of.

A few weeks ago, a small bump appeared above my lip. Once upon a time, I wouldn't have even noticed it, it's that tiny. But it's in the spot where some cancer cells still remain, and I've been warned to watch the area like a hawk. After losing a few nights of sleep, I finally got in to see the dermatologist. He's sure it's nothing, and on anyone else, he wouldn't give it a second thought. But I'm not anyone else. I am a melanoma survivor, and a rare and difficult to diagnose form at that, one that is known for recurring.

So the Hobsian choice. Biopsy and leave a visible scar above my lip? Or let it go for now and take a chance?

Poor Dr. Goldstein literally agonized over the decision. Not only did he not want to leave a scar, he also did not want to delay my starting work with UCLA on my nose, and doing a procedure now might have done just that.

He and Paul and I came to the conclusion that we would wait six weeks and revisit options then, of which there are several. In the meantime, over the next few weeks, I have my regular visits with the melanoma specialist and my oncological surgeon, so I'll have the benefit of several other opinions to weigh in.

The point in all this is that for many cancer survivors, it is never really over over. It's just over for now. There is always that lingering question, will my cancer come back? But it is a very important part of the process to learn to walk the tightrope of being vigilant for danger signs, but not constantly freaked out. Fortunately, I have a pretty good sense of balance, thanks to years of ballet, you know.

In the meantime, I just had my six-month CT scan to reconfirm that no nasty little cancer cells made it into the rest of my body. Won't have those results for a bit yet, but I'm not worried.

In fact, let me turn this whole entry back into the light, because that's really where my head is right now. I'm not worried about the silly little bump. It will be dealt with one way or another. I'm not worried about the CT scan. I'm not really worried about anything right now.

I'm looking forward to what will be, if not the actual end, the effective end of the road – my new nose.

That corny-ass expression about tomorrow being the first day of the rest of your life? Well, I'm definitely in the mood for some corn!

On a final note, I recently read through a lot of my early journal entries and realized how truly far I've come from the very beginning. There was a lot of anticipation then as well, but it was always for the scary stuff – anticipation before the surgery, before the bandages came off, before the tumor board's recommendation, before viability of implants was confirmed.

This time the anticipation is for something much desired. I'm whistling a lot these days. And it feels wonderful!

It's been a long time comin.'

Ignorance Really Is Bliss

January 19, 2012, 2:55 p.m.

If I only knew then what I know now. But thank goodness I didn't!

In our last episode, you may recall I was so excited about seeing Dr. Kelly at UCLA to start my nose that I could barely contain myself. What I did not know was that my session with him would turn out to be one of the most painful steps in the whole months-long process.

Losing a nose? Piece of cake. Implant surgery? No picnic, but bearable. Root canal? A walk in the park.

But removing the healing caps from the implants? Oh ... my ... God! Poor Paul barely has a hand left, I squeezed it so hard. Hurt like a sonofabitch. Once they got the healing caps off, then they had to screw on a temporary apparatus so they could take a mold. Also not fun.

Then they poured stinky liquid rubber on my face – which I smelled the remainder of the day – then slathered plaster over it, and I had to sit, completely motionless, for twenty minutes.

The whole experience was painful and unpleasant, but if that's what it takes to get a nose, then so be it. I'm just glad I did not know going in, so I didn't have to worry about facing something so painful.

OK, now that that's over, on to the good stuff. The next two sessions will be about sculpting – yay!!! This is the fun part, the part where I get to refine the look of my final nose. So it will still be my nose, but better! I think.

All in all, it was an exhausting day – physically because of the pain involved, emotionally because, well, for obvious reasons. But it's one more step I can check off the list, and there are fewer and fewer remaining. Dr. Kelly promised the worst was over. It was interesting that it did not hurt when they screwed the healing caps back on at the end, and they did not screw them on tightly, so they will have less trouble getting them off next time around.

At the end of it all, I wanted to do just one thing, hit Nate 'n Al's Deli for matzo ball soup and cheese blintzes, and that was exactly what we did. Nothing like good Jew food to soothe the pain.

Anyway, this isn't a particularly clever or thought-provoking entry, but I got yelled at by a few people for leaving everyone hanging by not reporting in. I had a really long work day yesterday, and just didn't have time to write. Apparently, there's a few Caring Bridge addicts out there. Better me than heroin or tobacco, I guess?

Next UCLA stop? One week on January 26.

A Very Short Story

January 23, 2012, 9:35 p.m.

Well, it finally happened. I came home from a lunch date with my dear friend, Esther, and took off my TFN – Temporary Fake Nose, for you newcomers. I was home only about 45 minutes when I realized I had to run a very quick errand.

It was pouring rain, which is no big deal in most places, but the end of the world to Los Angeles drivers. I threw on my jacket, grabbed my car keys and umbrella, raced out the door and hopped into my car. I had driven all the way down the block when I suddenly realized ...

I FORGOT TO PUT ON A NOSE!!!

I can't tell you how many times I am about to leave the house and stop myself at the last minute when I realize I forgot to put on my nose. This time, I was in such a hurry, it never even occurred to me that I didn't have one on.

I'm pretty sure my neighbor saw me through the window, and two other people were standing right next to my driveway as I pulled out. I can't imagine what they thought. My neighbor knows what happened, but hasn't ever seen me without a nose.

I turned the car around the minute I realized it, came home and stuck the TFN back on, but I wondered, what would have happened if I had shown up at the store with the big, fat hole in my face?

Hmmm, food for thought.

Survival

January 31, 2012, 9:35 p.m.

Whenever I suffer the loss of a loved one, these lyrics from a very old YES song come to mind:

> *"Don't doubt the thought there's life within you,*
> *Yesterday's endings will tomorrow life give you.*
> *All that dies, dies for a reason*
> *To put its strength into the season ... survival."*

The past week or so has been one of intense emotions – heartbreaking loss, enormous relief and tremendous elation. I am wrung out, exhausted with crying, tears of both sadness and joy.

Many of you know that Bailey, our beloved old cat, has been ill. Last Wednesday, we gave him a peaceful exit from this world, right here in our living room with the help of our very compassionate vet, Dr. Monica Revel. I've had many cats in my life, but he was so unique, so special and so much a part of our lives for over 16 years that we feel his loss deeply.

Many of you don't know that Bailey had only three legs. Yet of all the cats with whom I've shared my life, I cannot think of one who was more full of life and energy. He did everything with great vigor. And when he played, he played all out despite his missing leg. When he slept, it was the most sound sleep you could imagine. When he loved, his purr was louder than a Harley with no muffler. When he ate, he ate with such gusto we used to joke they could hear him smacking his lips all the way across the street.

And yet, it was his time. His cancer had spread, he was no longer the Bailey we knew. Life for him, and for us in caring for him, had become a struggle. So as hard it was to say goodbye, it was also a relief, for him even more than us.

The very next day after letting him go, we were back at UCLA to proceed with the creation of my prosthesis. But the joy of seeing myself with my new nose juxtaposed with the fresh pain of losing Bailey was confusing, to say the least. My heart was completely torn.

Now fast forward to yesterday's visit to the melanoma specialist, still less than a week after losing Bailey. First, Dr. Galani is certain the little bump above my lip is nothing to worry about, we will just keep an eye on it over the years. But he has declared me cancer free! My CT scans, my blood work, the physical exam he gave me – all clean, all clear, the best, happiest news one could ask for. I will live, hopefully, for a very long time.

Death ... and life. Two opposite sides of the coin. This may sound very weird to say, but I almost felt like Bailey let go of his life so that I could have mine, like he "took the bullet" for me.

He is gone and I am here.

And now, I feel free, released, like all the bad stuff is truly behind me, at least this round of bad stuff anyway. I've lost my nose, I've lost my Bai, but I've gained my life.

There have been a number of times in my life where I've felt as though I've completed a phase and am embarking on a new journey. One such time was when I met Paul and my single days were over. Not coincidentally, my beloved 20-year-old cat died just three weeks after Paul and I met. Letting go of Greta then allowed me to be free to start a new life with Paul and adopt two more cats, Bailey and Amanda.

"All things die for a reason, to put their strength into the season."

Bailey has put his strength into my new season, a new phase of my life and whatever it may bring. He lived his life full-out and, in that, he left me example of what I must now do to honor him.

I am well, I will live. And to honor Bailey, I must play as hard as I can, sleep as soundly as I can, love unabashedly, purr as loudly as I can, and eat with great gusto.

I owe him that.

Welcome Back, My Friends, To The Show That Never Ends

February 17, 2012, 10:19 p.m.

"Come inside, the show's about to start
Guaranteed to blow your head apart,
You've got to see the show, it's a dynamo
You've got to see the show, it's rock and roll!"

Yes, folks, life is rock and roll these days!

OK, so the rest of Emerson, Lake and Palmer's lyrics may not be so apropros to the situation, especially the part about the seven virgins and the mule, but this chorus just felt like what I wanted to say after such a long absence from you all.

Said absence, by the way, was thanks in part to my computer being in the shop for over a week, my getting yet another cold, working like crazy when I've been well to make up for all the times when I haven't been and, finally, a lovely bout with food poisoning the other night. It was mild, thank goodness. All of this was while still recovering from the painful final weeks of January.

I become nearly apoplectic if I allow myself to dwell on the ridiculous amount of stuff that has gone awry in the last few months. If I were to attempt to catalogue them here, it would become bigger than a volume of "Harry Potter."

Yet, as hard as it all has been – and it has, indeed, been hard – I still have the glorious emotional lift each week of visiting my new best friend and Minnesota homey, Dr. Kelly at UCLA.

No matter how stupid the rest of the week is, every week I'm like a kid that's waiting for a new toy. Picture

"Build-A-Bear," only it's "Build-a–Nose." Let me tell you, the process of creating my nose is fascinating, with painstaking care given to every detail.

It is also, at times, excruciatingly painful, and yes, I've learned to take Vicodin every week before I go.

The amazing thing is that when they put the nose on, I think it looks great. But Dr. Kelly, along with the sculptor – her name is Tomome, and she's incredible at what she does, has a very warm heart, and a wonderful smile – they see the flaws that even Paul and I don't notice. They tinker with it, put it back on, and voila' – it's magically even better!

We're coming to the end of the sculpting process, though, after much back-and-forth with the bottom of the nose to try to hide my scar, and yet not inhibit the move-ment of my upper lip. They are literally adding and taking away millimeters of wax trying to get it just right. Once the silicon is cast – that's it – no more tinkering. So they want the wax mold to be absolutely perfect.

Yesterday, they held up color samples to my face to try to determine what to use as a base. I understand the paint-ing can be the most difficult part as they try to perfectly match your skin tone. It's the last process and takes several visits.

Yesterday, they also brought in the final apparatus that is actually going to be screwed onto my implants. It's white gold, and I'm SO bloody excited, I could scream (in a good way), because in two weeks, they will put it on and leave it on permanently! No more pinching skin and pressing den-tal nerves as they screw it on each week. I've even posted a picture of that, so those of you that are squeamish, well, sorry, too bad, just don't look.

Finally, I would say the most amazing thing of all – except that it's all so amazing that I can't really say which part is most amazing – is that when they snapped the wax nose onto the apparatus, I could feel how secure it will be. In fact, when we were done, I forgot I was wearing it and was ready to put my coat on and leave with it on.

I can tell you, when I have my TFN taped on to my face, I never forget it's there. I'm conscious of it every minute. To have something on my face that I don't feel every second – nothing short of a miracle!

I am concerned about only one thing. There is so much build-up for the whole thing, I worry that when I get the actual silicon nose itself, will it live up to my expectations? I can't imagine it won't, but I think you can all understand my apprehension. How many times have you gone to a movie everyone raved about, only to think it was just "eh" because your expectations were so high?

I only know that I've lived through cancer, implant surgery, a root canal, sinus infections, the death of our cat, not to mention months of worries and fears about each step I took. Whether it's true or not, when I put that nose on my face and wear it out the door for the first time, I want to truly leave all the massive amounts of shit behind me.

A lot of the "shit" of recent months has been normal stuff that everybody deals with. Everyone loses beloved pets. Everyone gets root canals. Everyone struggles with getting sick. It just that every little thing has seemed SO much bigger because I'm doing it all without a nose.

I think I'm used to not having a nose. But then sometimes I pause and think – I DON'T HAVE A FUCKING NOSE!!!

I know when I get my prosthesis, it won't really be a magic bullet that fixes everything. But it will go a long, long, long way in making the rest of life easier to bear.

And we're only weeks away.

Who Are You Now?

March 1, 2012, 7:42 p.m.

It's the question of the hour that comes from an old obscure song from the Broadway version of Funny Girl – it never made it to the big screen. There's a verse:

> *"I know I am better, braver and surer too*
> *But who are you now?"*

Of course, Fanny Brice is talking to her lover. I'm talking to my nose, but it still feels apt. If anyone would understand my torturing the metaphor here, surely Barbra would.

You see, today I saw my almost-finished nose. I know that ultimately, I will be so thrilled to have it. But there's a longer emotional process to get there than I'd expected.

First, I have to face one scary fact. My prosthetic, for better or worse, is as good as it's going to get. All this time, living with my TFN, I've been able to comfort myself with the idea that something so much better is coming.

But with the prosthetic, we're done. There is no next step. And today, I realized (once again) that I am never again going to look the same as I did. I will look good (I hope), but the face I see in the mirror will be not be the face I've been looking at for so many years. The best prosthetic in the world still isn't my nose.

Please don't misconstrue this as ingratitude. Believe me, I'm so thankful that on March 15, I will be able to walk out into the world with something on my face that looks reasonably like a real nose. But there is a difference between a nose and my nose.

I remember feeling this way after I got my nose done almost 20 years ago. Even though it was by choice, even though it was a better nose than I was born with, there was a real adjustment period before I felt comfortable looking in the mirror.

This time around, it isn't by choice and it's good, but it isn't better, which makes the adjustment that much harder.

On an intellectual level, the process has been absolutely fascinating. Today, when they snapped on the final silicon nose before it was painted, it was a flat color and looked like a lifeless hunk. Then Tomome worked her magic for 20 minutes or so, painting and painting and painting with her little pallet, and when she was done – oh my God – what a transformation! Suddenly, the hunk of silicon had personality. Our skin is not a single flat color, and I don't know how she manages to create the illusion of actual skin, but she did.

We had a picture of my nose from before the surgery. I showed her my freckle I'd had for a gazillion years and asked if she could paint it on. She said, in her broken Japanese accent, pointing to the melanoma – you want all of these spots? No! I said, and tried to explain the other, bigger, blacker spots were the cancer, and I certainly did not want those back! We all had a good laugh and then she painted on the single tiny brown freckle. At first it was too low, so she simply painted over it and made it higher. What a bizarre process!

There are a few more things for Tomome to do; there's some kind of glaze and white powder she puts on it to make it look shiny in the places where skin naturally reflects, and matte in the places where you don't want it to shine, so the nose I saw today is not the final product.

On the 15th, Dr. Kelly will also paint the second nose. Tomome does one, he does the other – not sure why, which won't be finished for another two weeks. But I only need one nose to be "ready for my close-up, Mr. DeMille!"

I know it will take time for me to adjust to all this. It feels like so much to process right now. I also know that, once I'm used to it, I will go on about my merry way and eventually give it very little thought.

Beth Altman Pfeiffer, a brave cancer survivor who is machatunim – family by marriage, for those of you who don't speak Yiddish – once wisely advised me that a time would come when cancer and losing my nose would not be the first thing I think about when I wake up in the morning or the last thing I think about before falling asleep. I didn't really believe her when she said it, but after months had passed, I finally realized she was right.

Well, I have to trust her wisdom again, and believe that there will come a day when looking different will not be the first thing I think about when I look in a mirror.

But I'm not there just yet. Right now, I'm grieving all over again – hopefully for the last time – for the nose I had and lost.

La Ti Da, Ti Da

March 3, 2012, 8:08 p.m.

"Things are finally going swell,
The sun is shining, I'm feeling well
My mind is clear and finally,
I feel the happy coming back to me ...

So I sing la ti da, ti da, and I say la ti da, ti da ..."

Thanks to The Icicles for the cheeriest little ditty ever to grace commercial television. Sorry for the long intro, but the lyrics say it all today.

After a day or two of soul-searching and staring repeatedly – and I mean repeatedly – at photos Paul took at UCLA on Thursday of my almost-finished nose, "I've grown accustomed to my face."

I keep getting reminded that this is all a process. There are a multitude of conflicting feelings about every step, and sometimes I just have to wait until the dust settles before I understand how I really feel about something.

The more I look at those photos, the more I can't wait to get that nose. I have never looked perfect, so why should I expect that now? I don't want perfect, I don't need perfect. I need something that will make people see past the mess in the middle of my face to me – and no, I don't mean all of you wonderful friends and family – I mean all the strangers on the street, the clerk at the grocery store, the clients I meet every day, and mostly, every single little kid who stares unabashedly at the strange-looking lady with the weird thing on her face.

Once I get that nose, I hope my eyes and smile will become the first thing people notice about me. They have always been my "calling card," and I will be so happy when they are, once again, the most noticeable thing about me.

On a slight tangent of good news: I had another mole removed from my leg. Had it for a gazillion years, but it started to look a little different, so we lopped it off. Got the biopsy results yesterday – benign at the moment, but it did contain "atypical" cells, meaning if we had left it alone, it might have become trouble. So good riddance! Now I'm all clean again.

With that final boost, I'm past the doldrums of my prior entry. I may still have some hard moments ahead looking in the mirror, but I am now confident those moments will become more fleeting as time passes.

And once again, I have to say thanks to my wonderful Aitchy. When I told him this morning I was feeling much better about my new nose and was actually excited again, he just smiled and said, "I knew you'd get there." But he never pushed me, didn't try to minimize how badly I felt or stop my tears. He just let me be where I needed to be when I needed to be there and had faith in me that I would come to a better place in my own good time. Gotta love that man of mine.

So I sing:

"la ti da, ti da ..."

Countdown

March 11, 2012, 6:46 p.m.

Three more days. Three ... more ... days!

Just to put this in perspective for you all: It's been 276 days since I've been able to look in the mirror and see a whole face unobstructed by some concoction of tape and bandages. It's hard to remember what it's like to see myself.

As much as I like to think I'm used to the hole in my face, from a physical standpoint, there are times when it still feels uncomfortable and unnatural, and my prosthesis won't change that. But there are many things it will change.

Here are the ones I'm most looking forward to:

1.) I can't wait to blend into the crowd, for heads not to turn when they see me, no more double-takes, pitying looks or children's unabashed stares.

2.) I can't wait to not have to say to a new client, "please excuse the mess in the middle of my face, I'm just dealing with some medical issues, but I'm absolutely fine."

3.) I can't wait to not have tape on my face every day.

4.) I can't wait – seriously, I cannot wait – until I don't have to allot an extra 10 minutes to making a new nose in the morning. I don't do well in the morning as it is.

5.) I can't wait to not feel insecure about whether my nose is going to fall off. Just today, I tried on a shirt at the Gap, and when I put it on over my head, it caught on the top edge of my TFN and just about pulled the whole damn thing off.

And yet, even with all that I have to look forward to, I'm nervous and more than a little freaked out. Life is going to change, yet again. For the better, I assume, but change is rarely easy or without repercussions.

There is so much I've learned in this past year, yet nothing I've been through has quite prepared me for Thursday morning when I walk away from Dr. Kelly's office wearing my new nose – well, one of my new noses. I don't get the second one until April 3.

Which brings up another interesting question that can plague one in the wee hours of the morning when a hot flash wakes you. What if I like the placement of one nose better, but the paint job on the other nose better? How will I decide which one I prefer to wear?

Sound silly? You try choosing between fake body parts.

Anyway, all my questions will be answered in good time. And you know when they are, I will share it all right here.

One Day More

March 14, 2012, 7:30 p.m.

"Another day, another destiny ..."

This song that ends Act One of Les Miserables has always made me cry, and now, being in the mood to cry a lot, it felt perfectly suited for this post.

I cannot account for my constant desire to weep today. Maybe it's being so close to the end and the relief that entails. Maybe it's the fear that I won't be happy with the prosthetic.

Maybe it's the idea that I will be happy with the prosthetic and the tears will be those of joy. Maybe it's thinking about how much I love and cherish my Aitch, and all that he has meant to me and done for me this past year (and always), and how I could never (and I mean never) have survived this with my spirit intact without him.

For whichever of these reasons (or all), I am in a highly emotional place.

Today, when I got home from meeting with a client, I purged my bathroom of all the nose-making accoutrements that have cluttered the counter. I had no less than three boxes of different kinds of bandages, cloth tape, two different kinds of scissors, a template I created so I could cut a consistent shape each day, not to mention the three plastic noses themselves.

They are gone now, history – closed up and tucked away in a cabinet – out of sight, out of mind. I surveyed the newly spacious counter in my bathroom and felt a fresh sense of order. The end of the chaos.

To paraphrase the lyrics ...

> *"One day to a new beginning,*
> *raise the flag of freedom high!"* (flag = nose)

It seems appropriate to reflect again on all the stages I've been through this year; all the questions, and how every time a question was answered, it was followed by another question.

And how lucky I was with each answer. Yes, they got all the cancer. No, I did not need radiation. Yes, I could get the implants. Yes, the implants "took" well and healed properly. Yes, the prosthetic would be covered by Kaiser.

All the right things had to happen to reach this day, and they did. Only one question remains, and it will be answered tomorrow.

Besides the terror and elation, I'm feeling my favorite thing to revel in: A great, big, fat, heaping dose of gratitude for having reached this point in the journey. The end of the tunnel. Time to step out of the darkness and into a life of endless possibilities.

> *"Tomorrow we'll discover*
> *what our God in heaven has in store!*
> *One more dawn, One more day, One day more!"*

Disappointment Sucks

March 15, 2012, 3:23 p.m.

No nose today after all. I am in meltdown mode and don't really want to talk about it, but wanted to let you all know, since you were expecting to hear something exciting.

Will post when I'm ready to resurface.

Sorry, guys.

Time to Pick Myself Up, Dust Myself Off

March 16, 2012, 5:12 p.m.

Well, you know the rest.

So now that I've had 24 hours to absorb the blow of yesterday, here's the story:

Yesterday at UCLA, we began by trying on the second nose so it could be painted. Lo and behold, the second nose actually feels like an even better fit – just by a hair's breath, but it seemed slightly more "intimate," to borrow Dr. Kelly's lingo. Dr. Kelly painted most of it, then Tomome took over (in part, we think, because Dr. Kelly was taking so long). All in all, I actually think I like the second nose a bit better.

Then I waited eagerly for my first nose to be brought in and put on me, which is when Dr. Kelly informed me that the final glaze they put on it just hadn't "cured" completely, it was still a bit tacky to the touch, and they did not feel it I should wear it until it's completely dry.

You know the saying about your heart dropping into your stomach? Mine didn't do that. It felt more like my heart had dropped onto the floor where everyone was stomping on it.

Now, looking at this from a rational perspective, I only have to wait another week for my nose. This does not seem like such a big deal, right?

Wrong. So wrong.

Yes, it's only a week. But I have been hanging on by my fingernails for so long now, it seems I don't have the strength to last even one more day, let alone a week.

It was this setback that showed me how fragile I still am, how much it has taken out of me to present myself to the world every day.

And suddenly, it wasn't about waiting another week for the prosthetic.

I was in such a bad state, I couldn't even share it with my Aitch. I had to shut myself in the bedroom and cut loose with the full hideous depth of grieving for my nose, wishing in a way I had never allowed myself before, that I hadn't lost it in the first place – privately lamenting the whole horrible freak show this year has been. And knowing full well the probability that even when I get this Holy Grail of a prosthetic, it will still just be a fake nose! And finally, being exhausted with being "brave and inspiring" and patient and grateful and all those things have kept me going till now.

I haven't been terribly angry since this all this began last year. I'm not, by nature, an angry person, and anger often seems like such a wasteful and negative use of energy. But yesterday (and even now), I was/am angry that I have yet another hoop to jump through.

I don't have the strength for even one more hurdle. I'm at the point where I just want life to be fucking easy for a change! It doesn't seem like so much to ask.

And yet, that's just not how life works.

Here's where I usually think about how much harder so many people have it, and how lucky I am that it's only my nose, and that I'm cancer-free, etc.

But I'm not in my usual place and I don't feel lucky right now. I feel like someone who has suffered an enormous loss from which I will never completely recover.

Of course, that's today – OK, and probably tomorrow and for a few more days, at least until Thursday.

This depressed, angry, impatient place is not a natural

place for me to be. It's not a comfortable place for me to be. I prefer feelings of blessedness and gratitude. But right now, this is where I am, and I just have to sit with it for the moment.

This morning, I had to get up and go to work. I had to pull out all the band-aids and tape and crap that I had tucked away, so I could put a new TFN together. I did it because I had to, because that's what you do.

But believe me, if I could have my druthers, I would crawl into bed, pull the covers over my head for a week-long sob-fest, and not come out until next Thursday at 9 a.m.

Life has to go on, though. Hiding is not really a choice. So, I'll just keeping picking myself up and dusting myself off, but I won't really be "starting all over again" until that new nose is on my face – and maybe not even then.

Thanks to all of you for your kindness and empathy. It is certainly appreciated.

People Who Need People

March 17, 2012, 9:35 p.m.

Lesson for the day: There's a reason why we should not isolate ourselves for any extended period of time. A day or two to wallow, OK. But here's what happens when you spend too much time hiding away – you completely lose perspective.

In our last chapter, you all know I really wanted to spend the week hibernating in the safe seclusion of my home. Today, before seeing a client, I had to run an errand – had to – even though it was cold and blustery and rainy and nasty and I would have given anything not to leave the house at all.

But an interesting thing happened. While making my way through the hustle and bustle of The Grove (our nearby outdoor mall, for those of you who are not in L.A.), I crossed paths with a young woman in a wheelchair being pushed by a young man. The thought that immediately ran through my head was, "Thank God I can walk! What would I do if I weren't ambulatory?"

In that instant, I stopped feeling angry and depressed about the week's delay of my nose delivery.

Please know, this was not a conscious attempt to get into a different head space, it was a natural reaction I had to seeing someone who seemed to be worse off than me.

And when I realized that, I understood why barricading yourself alone in your own private space isn't really a good idea for more than a brief respite.

Humanity is out there for a reason – we are meant to be a part of it, to be part of the collective. People will annoy us,

amuse us and amaze us – and some we will take no notice
of at all. But John Donne said it much better than I ever
could and several parts of "No man is an island" have been
often quoted. But one line you never seem to hear quoted
that I felt quite strongly today:

"... *I am involved in mankind.*"

And I am so much the better for it. Thursday will come
soon enough.

P.S. (and maybe I should have led with this) Also while
at The Grove, a homeless guy wolf-whistled at me!
Go figure.

Silent Night, Noseless Night

March 21, 2012, 11:20 p.m.

"I am calm, but wish I were tight" (to paraphrase)

I am oddly relaxed tonight. I was so deflated at the aborted nose delivery last week, that I seem completely dispassionate tonight about the fact that I will likely get it tomorrow.

Yup, tomorrow should be the day. But I don't take anything for granted anymore.

As Paul and I always say about our respective businesses when we think a meeting has gone well, but we have not closed: "It doesn't mean anything until the check is in your hand."

Well, in this case, nothing means anything until the nose is on my face.

Maybe tomorrow?

Could be. Who knows? OK, no mixing West Side Story and Christmas carols – it just ain't right.

Say goodnight, Gracie.

Speechless in Los Angeles

March 22, 2012, 9:35 p.m.

I feel like I want to share the day with you all, but I have absolutely no idea what to say! A rarity for me. My emotions have run the entire gamut today, and I still have a lot of adjusting to do. So I'll just say this:

YES, I got my nose this morning. NO, it isn't perfect.

Of course, when I look in the mirror, I see all the flaws. It still looks like a fake nose to me. I see the borders quite clearly and markedly.

Paul, of course, thinks I look wonderful and I caught him staring at me and smiling at odd moments throughout the day.

Other people I know and encountered today seemed to think it looked just fine – even great. But insecurity and paranoia make me question their veracity.

I will say this: (a) it's a vast improvement; and (b) how good it looks depends entirely on the lighting I'm in. In sunlight, the color difference between the nose and my skin seems painfully apparent. In the light in my bathroom, not so much. In some light, at certain angles, it's barely noticeable.

In other words, it's all completely subjective and malleable and I will need quite some time to wrap my head around the whole thing.

My initial reaction this morning was to feel enormously insecure walking out of UCLA with it on. I felt like the whole world could see that I was wearing a fake nose. By tonight, as Paul and I walked out of the restaurant where we had dinner, I said to him, "How come nobody is looking at me?"

If he hadn't known I was playing, I think he would have slapped me upside the head. I must say there was a ridiculously huge drop in the number of stares I got being out in public. That, I think, is a good thing.

So, like everything else this past year – or basically in life – it's a process.

The best part of the day, I must admit, was discovering that The Counter (where we ate) serves "adult shakes." Read: a coffee malt with Kahlua. OMG! It's the greatest invention ever! Yummy, sweet and gives you quite the buzz. (And, yes, I'm still under the influence of said buzz.)

Anyway, the suspense is over. Now it's just a matter of getting used to the new me which is really just the old me with a hunk of silicone on my face.

I am curious and eager, though, to see how the second nose will compare, when I receive it on April 3.

Stay tuned.

F**kin' Perfect

March 27, 2012, 12:44 p.m.

"Pretty pretty please, don't you ever ever feel
Like you're less than fuckin' perfect"

Ah, my girl Pink says it for me once again. Five days in and I certainly have had an attitude adjustment.

No, the prosthesis is not perfect, but I've come to realize that if I was expecting to have a hunk of silicone clipped to my face and still look as though nothing had happened to me, then I was sadly delusional.

So I'm learning to let go of my delusions of probiscal grandeur (no, I don't know if that's actually a word, but it is now).

The first realization that lifted my spirits was the fact that when light and shadow hit the human face, it creates lines that aren't really there. My lines are actually there, but as everyone keeps telling me, other people don't notice them the same way I do.

So I started noticing them everywhere. I made Paul pause the TV the other night so I could point out the line created by the lighting on the side of Julianna Margulies' nose that runs almost exactly the same way the edge of my prosthesis runs.

My next and even more important realization was that shit happens to people's faces all the time.

People are scarred or burned or maimed in some way that means they will never be "perfect" again. And they all learn to live with their own imperfection. That is who I am now and acknowledging it means I can accept it in a way I had not done before.

A big, giant dose of perspective was also gifted me yesterday. I was at the hair salon and I picked up "People" magazine and while flipping through it, I landed on an article that stunned me and brought me to tears.

It was the story of Stephanie Nielson, a beautiful young woman and her handsome husband – until a plane crashed completely deformed her face (I mean horrific burn scars) and also scarred her husband.

This amazing, brave woman rose up, literally from the ashes – her body was 80 percent burned – and carried on with her life with joy and gratitude! You could see it in her eyes that she is happy just to be alive. This absolutely blew me away. She has a book coming out, "Heaven is Here."

Talk about perspective. My prosthesis is a work of art and beauty in comparison.

This doesn't mean I won't be self-conscious at times. This doesn't mean I won't still grieve my old nose. It only means that anytime I get too enmeshed in my own crap, I have something concrete to pull me out, and it's remembering this:

I am now one of those people with an imperfect face. I am Stephanie Nielson with the burn scars. I am Sandy Duncan with the fake eye. I am Tina Fey with the scar that men find oddly titillating. I am Lauren Scruggs, the model whose face was slashed by a helicopter blade. I am Marla Hanson, who had her face destroyed by some lunatic with a knife.

I am Barbara Caplan-Bennett with a prosthetic nose, and that's just fine and dandy, because I am still Barbara Caplan-Bennett! And I always kind of liked her.

Raise Your Glass

March 29, 2012, 8:37 p.m.

> *"If you are wrong in all the right ways*
> *All my underdogs, we will never be, never be*
> *Anything but loud and nitty gritty, dirty little freaks"*

Sorry, but I am so in a Pink mood these days. And yup, that's me, a dirty little freak!

Oh, stop gasping, I mean that in good-humored, joking, best way possible. I always used to say in my old hippie days, you don't want to be too normal, because then you're really weird. It's always better to be a little weird, because then you're actually normal.

Did you follow that? Remember, I said it first while indulging in some "herbal" smokeables back in the '70's.

Drug-induced logic notwithstanding, I still find the philosophy works for me. And so, it is with that belief system that I proudly fly my new freak flag nose. I even went to Century City shopping center today and did not turn a single head. That's a good thing.

I have had a few set–backs – e.g., someone I spent time with a few days ago (perhaps it was too soon) whose attitude did nothing to put me at ease with how I now look, but only made me more self–conscious. I am learning quickly who it is safe to spend time with and who it is not until I'm completely down with the whole thing.

But it's not someone else's job to make me feel OK with myself, it's mine. And in that regard, I'm mostly good. I've seen several clients already – even sold a job today.

Once I get going on a job site, I tend to forget about my face.

My friend, Kathrin, who has been at the ready with all sorts of good wisdom throughout this past year, said something that really made sense. She opined that when I stop physically feeling the nose on my face – which I will eventually, when I really get used to it – then I will lose my self-consciousness.

And I think she's absolutely right. As long as I can feel it, I think about it. But I feel it less and less, and eventually, it will be like my contact lenses – I'll forget it's even there.

This Saturday, I will be seeing a few dozen friends at a party, and frankly, I'm a little nervous. But I am ready and think it will be a good thing to jump into the pool with both feet. No toe-dipping allowed when you're amidst a group of dear friends, which they all are.

And I will be sure to raise my glass, because I am wrong in all the right ways.

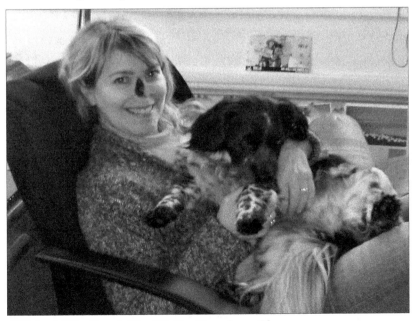

"Dirty Little Freak" in All My Noseless Glory

Only One Question Remains

April 16, 2012, 9:35 p.m.

And that question is ... now what?

Today was my last real appointment at UCLA. Dr. Kelly shaved off a few spots inside Nose No.1, so it now fits better, looks better and I can even breathe better. Amazing such a minor adjustment can make such a big difference.

Nose No. 2 looks slightly different, but I can't judge whether it's better or just different because it's not dry yet and I can't wear it for another week. More on it in the next (final?) post. But since Nose No.1 has been "fixed," I'm no longer waiting for Nose No. 2 with bated breath (no pun intended).

By the way, to avoid the "Nose 1 and Nose 2" business, I've decided to name my noses after the March sisters (from "Little Women" for the nonreaders among you, or for those of you with a Y chromosome.) The first is Meg, the second is Jo, and in a few years, when I need a replacement, it will be Beth. By the time I work my way through nose Amy, maybe they'll come up with a better solution than a clip-on prosthetic – but I'll cross that bridge when I come to it.

I will have to stop in at UCLA again at the end of April for some minor adjustments on Jo, but I think of today as being the official end of the line that began last spring.

April 27, 2011, I walked into the dermatologist's office and was told, "It's probably nothing, but we need to biopsy that." Do they always say "it's probably nothing" just so you don't freak out?

So here we are, almost a full year later. A year I've spent constantly running to doctor appointments, filling prescriptions, taking tests – so many tests – and waiting ... always endless waiting ... for answers to so many questions.

There are no more questions now. I am done. This is me and my new life, but just what exactly does that mean?

I feel a bit like Frodo at one of the five endings of "Return of the King" movie (an in-joke for LOTR fans).

Like Frodo, I've achieved my goal of saving my world from evil (cancer) with the help of my Sam-wise (Paul), I'm missing a body part (him a finger, me a nose), I'm a bit haggard from the journey, but was surrounded by loved ones at a party Saturday night for my official "return" to my life.

I was nervous about seeing all my closest friends at one time, and knowing that every one of them would be scrutinizing my prosthetic – judging it, being happy for me or pitying me, depending on whether they deemed it amazing or awful.

But it turned out to be a wonderful evening. People were kind and supportive and generous with compliments. It was just the spoonful of sugar I needed to leave all this behind me and walk forward into the world with my head held high. Which is exactly what I now must do.

But where am I going when I march forward? What am I to do now that I'm done with the business of healing?

Several answers come to mind.

The first is obvious and immediate. I've spent a year being completely self–absorbed, thinking only about me, me, me. But as Bette Midler said in "Beaches:" "Enough about me, what do you think of me?" (Jami, do you remember us seeing that together?) I always loved that line.

It's time to start thinking outside myself again. I have not volunteered at a single Best Friends event in a year. The big Super Adoption event is at the end of this month, and

Paul and I intend to be back at our old stations helping all the local rescue groups of Los Angeles find forever homes for hundreds of deserving dogs and cats. There's nothing that works quite so well at pulling you out of self-absorption as helping animals who can't help themselves.

Then, of course, there's "the book" everyone's been telling me I need to write. Frodo did that, too, if you recall. But I'm not quite ready to take that on yet. I have a vacation coming in May and a birthday in June. For now, I am giving myself permission to just kick back and enjoy life. On my 58th birthday, I will reassess and look towards making this past year mean something by turning these posts into a cohesive volume.

Then there's the whole "inspirational speaking" thing, and though I'd love to try to find a way to do that at some point down the road, again – just not ready. I think it will go hand-in-hand with working on a book.

Which brings me to the final "now what?" Do I keep posting here? There's really nothing to add to all I've said. My medical crisis is past – that journey is over, and what-ever new journeys I embark upon, this is not the appropriate forum for those.

I will check back in once or twice more over the next few weeks, because I don't know what surprises may come up with my new nose, or if I can quit cold turkey!

But posting here does have to come to an end, and I suspect it will be soon. I will sorely miss writing to you all, and will contemplate other, more appropriate places to blog.

But the one thing Frodo did, which I will not do, is sail off into the sunset with the elves, leaving his dearest and closest Hobbit friends behind. For without my amazing friends, and without so many wonderful people who have followed this blog, this journey would have felt empty and meaningless.

I know it's weird to think of having cancer as being a "meaningful" experience, but my connection with all of you via Caring Bridge has made it just that.

I always felt the three "Lord of the Rings" movies embodied many references and homages to my all–time favorite, "The Wizard of Oz," so instead of following Frodo's lead here and sailing away, I will follow Dorothy Gale's – surrounding myself with loved ones and saying, "There's no place like home!"

Cue the swell of music.

I've Grown Accustomed to My Face

April 22, 2012, 2:19 p.m.

And here we are, a year from where we began, and life finally, is back to normal (as Paul put it, whatever the hell that means).

Despite many people's assurances to the contrary, I still think it's quite obvious that I'm wearing a prosthetic nose. However, I have grown accustomed to the feel of it and there are so many ways in which it is a spectacular improvement over the TFN,

First, condensation no longer collects, so water doesn't spontaneously drip down my lip (a constant source of embarrassment – especially in front of clients).

And the prosthetic feels so secure, I never worry that it's going to fall off (a constant source of anxiety with the TFN).

Finally, if I pass you on the sidewalk, you'd have no idea there's something a bit "off" about me, as opposed to the obvious mess in the middle of my face with the TFN (a constant source of annoyance).

So take away the embarrassment, the insecurity and the annoyance, and it's all good. It's all good, of course, as long as I don't care if someone talking face-to-face with me can see that I'm wearing a prosthetic. And ya know what, I have – at long last – come to a place where I really don't give a flying rat's ass anymore.

Seriously – I have a prosthetic nose and so-fucking-what!?!?!?!

It makes me laugh to write this, because it's such a

relief not to care anymore. Look, once upon a time, I was a young, single woman with a hot dancer's body and lots of vanity about my looks.

But I am past my youthful vanity. I can't really pull off wearing a bikini anymore and the "waddle" on my neck is beyond the help of firming creams – yet my life is more gratifying than it ever was at 35 when I was closer to physical "perfection."

I'm racing toward 60 at the speed of light (OK, it's still two years away), I'm married to an amazing man who adores me, if I may be so bold as to put words into his mouth, I manage to still have considerable success designing and selling closets to strangers every day.

If my husband doesn't care, if my friends don't care, if my clients don't care – why the hell should I?

Let's see ... what are the five stages of grief again? Denial (check). Anger (check). Bargaining (check). Depression (check).

And the final step – Acceptance. I think I am ready to check this one off as well.

I know these stages aren't static. They come and go, but the moments when I feel loss are growing fewer and farther apart.

And the more I get my life back, the less I think about it.

Since I last posted, we attended two Dodger games. I had forgotten how wonderful and relaxing it is to sit in the stadium, facing the mountains on a glorious southern California day, watching a nail-biter that we managed to win in the final innings. My team is back on its feet, and Paul and I will be there to cheer them on.

More importantly, Best Friends Animal Society just launched an amazing program NKLA (No Kill L.A.) – to stop the euthanization of animals in the shelters. It's a massive program to reduce the number of pets killed in shelters in L.A. from 17,000 last year to ZERO! An ambitious endeavor, to be sure, but nothing changes without Herculean effort. And Paul and I are back involved just in time to be a part of it.

So life is very good. I have many years ahead of me, and I don't plan to spend a lot of time wringing my hands over my physical imperfections.

On a final note, I don't know why – and I could be quite literally dead wrong – but the other day, I was suddenly struck with the firm belief that my cancer is not coming back.

All precautions must still be taken. I'm on schedule with all my check-ups and another CT scan in July. But I firmly believe I am done. The statistical survival rate for Stage II melanoma is 80–20. Well, I plan to be in whatever percentage never sees their melanoma again. (B'li ayin hora! – or the Jewish version of "knock on wood" for those of you who are not familiar.)

So, from My Fair Lady to the Beatles ...

"Obla–di, obla–da,
life goes on, brah! ...
la la la how LIFE GOES ON!"

So Long, Farewell, Auf Wiedersehen, Goodbye

May 28, 2012, 3:11 p.m.

Something happened today, something wonderful, something that meant my life has come full circle and that this should be my final post.

But I'll save that story for the end.

First, let me say what an amazing vacation we had in South Florida. It was finally the stress-free vacation we'd been hoping for. Oh sure, the typical things went awry. The weather was not great, we got chewed up by jellyfish larvae swimming in the waters off of Key Largo (so itchy!), we got stuck in a plane on a runway waiting out a hail storm (nothing inspires confidence before takeoff like a hail storm) – you know, that kind of stuff.

But none of the little glitches overshadowed the enjoyment of the touring the Everglades via boat and tram, seeing alligators, turtles, unusual birds and natural beauty, visiting with dear cousins and a few old friends, having possibly the best fish meal ever at the Fish House in Key Largo, and the highlight of the trip, swimming with dolphins.

It was absolutely everything I would have done a year ago, before the whole nose debacle.

Everything.

I want to thank everybody here, once again, for being so incredibly supportive over the past year. You all gave me a softer landing than I ever could have had without you. Your encouragement, praise, empathy and advice were so appreciated.

Yes, I plan to do something with my story, but I'm still giving myself until my birthday in a few weeks to not worry about "doing" anything important.

In the meantime, I opened a blog page on Google entitled "On the Nose," but have not written anything yet. I will announce on Facebook when I start.

July 5 is the anniversary of my surgery, and I had actually planned to post here until then. But this brings me to what happened this morning that told me today would be the last entry.

Paul and I walked to breakfast at our favorite place (Toast on 3rd Street). On the way home, we passed a taco joint where people sit outside and eat. There was a family of six seated at the picnic table, and as we approached, I noticed the Mom staring at me with a quizzical expression.

As you all know, I'm quite used to being stared at, though it has rarely happened since I got my prosthetic. So I see her staring and I start wondering in my head, "Gee, I have a hat on and sunglasses and she is still staring! Is my fake nose really that obvious?"

"Excuse me!" she calls to us. I'm thinking, seriously? You're going to ask me about my nose?

She smiles, points to the NKLA t-shirt I'm wearing and says, "I've been seeing billboards all over town with a dog and the letters NKLA. What is "NKLA?"

I was THRILLED!!!! I love when people ask so I can tell anyone who will listen about "No Kill Los Angeles," the Best Friends program to end euthanasia of healthy, adoptable animals in the L.A. shelter system in the next five years.

I explained the program and she loved the idea. I gave her the website so she can get more info and donate.

It wasn't until we walked away that it really hit me

hard. It was the first time in a year that I was being stared at for the right reason – so I can share my passion of helping animals!

My life, once again, is really truly about something besides cancer.

And with that I can finally say, so long, farewell.

Happy Ending

June 2020

It's been nine years since I lost my nose, eight years since my last Caring Bridge entry. But my story wouldn't be complete without sharing what happened after I last posted.

For the first year, many people encouraged me to turn my Caring Bridge entries into a book, but honestly, I didn't want to dwell on it anymore. I had spent a year of my life thinking of nothing but cancer, prosthetics, and freakdom. By the time I wrote that last piece, I was ready to move on and not look back.

But now, all these years later, the Great Pandemic of 2020 has given me time to reflect on what I went through. I woke up one morning (in isolation with Paul) and realized I was ready. So for anyone who might want to know what life looked life after my last Caring Bridge post, this is how it went:

***   ***   ***

First, perhaps most important: I am still cancer free.

I see my surgeon, Dr. McNicoll, once a year, which Paul and I always enjoy because he likes to tell us stories.

I see Dr. Goldstein twice a year for a full body skin exam and he's cut more chunks off of me than I can count, but so far, only one had signs of becoming trouble, and he got it all. He still feels compelled to warn me that I'll have a scar every time he cuts something off, and we still laugh about it.

My current oncologist, Dr. Milani, sees me once a year to review my annual PET scan and blood work. And as much as I dislike the PET scan process (no carbs or sugar, i.e., no chocolate for 24 hours prior), there's a lot of comfort in knowing I'm still clean.

Recently, Dr. Milani shared with me the tremendous progress research has made with melanoma treatment. I asked him if I were diagnosed today, would I still have had to lose my nose? His answer? Very possibly not. They would try new treatments first.

Friends always make a sad face when I tell them this. "Doesn't it make you feel bad that you might not have had to lose your nose?" they ask. No, it doesn't. It makes me feel good, because it alleviates the single fear that has lived in the depths of my consciousness all these years – the fear of losing another piece of my face if my melanoma returns.

Knowing that "to cut is to cure" is no longer the only way to deal with melanoma is a huge relief.

I do believe, however, that after my tenth anniversary next year, everyone but Dr. Goldstein will cut me loose and send me off into the world hoping I will never have to see them again. And as much as I'll miss my docs, I'll be happy to hit that milestone.

*** *** ***

As for life without a nose, it's been an interesting progression to "normalcy."

First, I have to share that I still get phantom feelings and itches where my nose would be, even all these years later. They are infrequent at this point, but when it happens, it's a freaky sensation. I think I will probably have them the rest of my life.

As for my prosthetics – the original pair were good, but not great. I felt it was obvious I was wearing a prosthetic and their shape wasn't as close to my original nose as I had hoped. But I was so shell-shocked going through the process in that first year, I had no idea how to ask for what I wanted. I just wanted a nose – any nose – so I could go on with my life.

And go on with my life I did.

Paul and I adopted our dog, Cally. She had been left tied to a post at a gas station with a shattered leg. Animal control was called and she was taken to a nearby shelter where they were going to euthanize her.

Swooping in to save the day was our friend and animal rescue angel, Robin Harmon, who found funding for her surgery and a foster home for her recovery. Her foster mom was my Facebook friend through our rescue connections, and when we saw Cally's picture on one of her posts, we fell in love.

Our Girl had several names as she changed hands, but we named her Cally – a mash-up of Dr. Cassarino, the pathologist who saved my life by finding how deep my

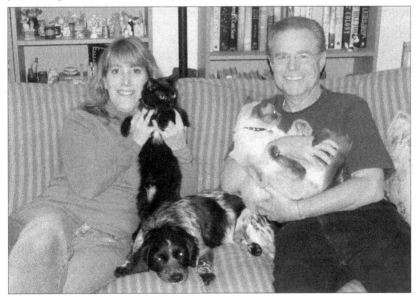

Our Little Family

cancer really went, and Dr. Kelly, the first prosthodontist who gave me my face back.

Paul and I took her everywhere we went and in that first year especially, when I was still self-conscious, Cally was great at diverting attention from my face. Who doesn't want to pet a friendly, adorable dog? It was amazing how much that helped me brave facing the world.

And just as important, if not more so, she became the light of Paul's life – something he needed and so deserved after being my caregiver and rock for so long.

So we are now a family of five, me and Paul, Cally, and of course, William and Beckett, the cats, still rule the roost. Our home is a happy one, where no one cares whether I have a nose or not.

*** *** ***

Of course, I went back to work at Closets By Design, where Jose, John and Mary were, as they always had been, accommodating in how they eased me back into full-time work.

But out in the field meeting clients, it was just me alone facing the music. I was no longer wearing the plastic taped on monster that was so obvious that it provoked immediate comment. So, when I'd arrive at a new client's home, I was still keenly aware of their reaction to seeing me for the first time. Could they tell I was wearing a prosthetic? Did they notice something was different about my face? I couldn't help but wonder what they thought.

Most people did not have an obvious reaction, yet I felt compelled at some point during the hours I spent with them to comment on the fact that I wore a prosthetic nose.

An old friend who was a psychologist once told me

I have a "disclosure complex," meaning I feel the need to tell everyone everything. I guess the sheer fact that I'm writing this book is proof that he was correct! Well, for better or worse, I felt the need to disclose to my clients what had happened to my face. Of course, I didn't just blurt it out. I always waited for an appropriate segue to bring it up.

And sharing my story often prompted clients to share theirs. I was shocked to hear how many people knew someone close to them who had battled melanoma – many who hadn't survived.

And if I didn't mention it myself, a few clients actually asked me in a very respectful way if I'd had skin cancer. Those were always people who knew someone who'd had surgery to remove cancer from their face and now fear being in public because they are scarred. Those clients wanted to know my story so they could share it with their loved one to help them feel less like a freak.

Of course, there were *those* people, a handful of clients who were horrible. One guy answered his door, pointed at my face, and said, "what's goin' on there with your nose?" One man asked in a rude tone if I was wearing "those allergy strips." A few people just stared unabashedly but without addressing the elephant in the room. They just stared.

But almost without fail, complete strangers were kind and empathetic, which I so appreciated.

$$*** \quad *** \quad ***$$

I should mention here how lucky I was to be able to get the implant that I so fretted over. Putting on and taking off my noses is a simple click, like snapping something into place. I knew if I couldn't have the implant, and was forced to glue my nose on, it would have made my life much more complicated. But back then, I could not have foreseen that early in the process, just how big of a deal it would be.

I change noses throughout the day like most women change outfits. I wear my second-best nose for work (because I'm exposed to sawdust and drywall mud and other hazards). When I come home, I swap to an old nose to take the dog for a walk. Then, if we're getting together with friends, I switch that out for my best nose. None of that would be possible if I were gluing on my nose each time. The sheer process of applying the glue, then cleaning it off later is time-consuming.

But the worst part is that I don't think I would ever have felt completely secure in wearing something glued to my face. I cannot say how many times throughout the past nine years I've thanked God, the fates and the universe that I was able to get my implant!

*** *** ***

As the years passed, my first pair of noses aged. Their edges frayed, their color faded and eventually it was time to go through the process of getting new prosthetics. Back to UCLA and Dr. Kelly we went. This time, the process was shorter because the preliminary work with my implant had already been done. It was only about making the nose itself.

And I was more prepared. I asked for more changes and they sculpted the wax mold until I thought I was satisfied. The end result was a better, more natural shape. Still not exactly "me," but definitely an improvement.

And the bonus? While Paul and I were meeting with Dr. Kelly, he showed us a book that contained his research paper about facial prosthetics that had been published in the U.K., in which my case was cited! So somewhere in Great Britain, young doctors are staring at my picture and reading about me. Not exactly my dream of how to get my 15 minutes of fame, but I'll take it!

Unfortunately, that visit also brought the news that Dr. Kelly was leaving UCLA to head up the Maxillofacial Department at Mayo Clinic. My homey was returning to Minnesota, and good for him! But so not good for me.

What would happen when I needed my next set of noses?

How would anyone be as good at what he does or as kind in working with us?

Enter Dr. Jay Jayanetti! I returned to UCLA in 2017 for my third set of noses with great trepidation, but my fears were completely unfounded. Not only was Dr. Jay incredibly good at the technical part of creating a new nose, the man was a bona fide artist. Paul and I watched with fascination as he took an old photograph of me and used it to shape the wax the way Michaelangelo might have used a model to sculpt The David. (OK, a little hyperbole perhaps.)

Of course, it didn't hurt that he was incredibly young and handsome. Being an old lady, I felt completely free to flirt shamelessly with him – yes, even in front of Paul, who knew well what I thought of my "hot doc." It also didn't hurt that he was extremely kind, and also just an interesting human being.

Fast forward to now – I'm the proud owner of four sets of noses. I ran out of March sisters as namesakes after the two sets (Meg, Jo, Beth and Amy), so the third set was named for the eldest Bennet sisters from Pride and Prejudice – Jane and Elizabeth.

The last set Dr. Jay made for me a year ago – Charlotte and Emily (Bronte) – are nothing short of spectacular. I finally learned exactly what I wanted and how to ask for it, and he was artist enough to be able to give it to me. My current set of noses are the closest I've come to looking like I did before my rhinectomy.

As I've said before, nothing is perfect. But I certainly couldn't come any closer! Finally – FINALLY – I can look in the mirror and see ME. The sheer joy and relief that comes with that is indescribable. When I'm out in public, I rarely give a thought to the fact that I'm wearing a fake nose.

The fun and benefit of now having old noses is that I wear them for "high risk" behavior, like being out in the sun or exercising, or even going to the dentist. And just like Eleanor Rigby, I keep a nose in a drawer by the door so it's handy when someone comes knocking.

*** *** ***

So what have I lost in the process? Not much! Swimming is still an issue because putting my head under water means it rushes into my the empty space and I feel like I'm being waterboarded. For a while I tried different ways to seal it off, but nothing really worked.

Then, during the creation process of my second set of noses, one of them developed a flaw and Dr. Kelly offered it to me unpainted, since they were just going to throw it away. I turned that into my "swimming nose."

It helps immensely and I can go underwater briefly, breathing out to keep the water from rushing in. Still, in short order, water starts to seep into around the edges.

But let's face it, I was never planning to be Mark Spitz. I can still enjoy a pool or lake in a limited way, and it's good enough. If this is the worst thing I suffer from surviving cancer, well, I can live with that.

***   ***   ***

Otherwise, life is as "normal" as it gets. I go to work, we go to the movies, play poker, have game night, travel. Basically, Paul and I do all the things we always did. When I arrive home from being out for the day, the first thing I do is take off my bra (like many women) and my nose (like no women).

My social life is pretty much exactly what it was in the "before" days. Right after I got my first set of noses, I had a small coming-out party so all my friends could see me for the first time with my prosthetic. It was just easier for me to face them all at once than to go through it over and over.

I knew some of my friends were fascinated by what was under my prosthetic and others were extremely squeamish and could not bear the thought of what I must look like without my nose. In order to satisfy the curiosity of the former, but not horrify the latter, I made an announcement. Anyone who wanted to see what I looked like without my nose, should follow me to the bedroom.

With a group of about seven or eight people watching, I removed my prosthetic and let everyone peer into the hole in my face. People oohed and aahed, amazed to see what's inside everyone's head. They also were curious about the implanted mechanism to which I clip my noses. This may sound perverse, but it was actually fun! I like when people find it fascinating. I like that people are curious. I like answering all their questions. (The first question is always, can you still smell things? The answer is a resounding yes!)

Something about being an object of fascination makes the whole thing more palatable. I'm a source of interest rather than disgust.

And for those who are very squeamish, I understand.

I'm not offended. I'm not upset.

But here's the beauty of it all. I've become so accustomed to my face without a nose that it's led to some pretty funny episodes.

The best example happened on Passover, about four years after the Great Nose Debacle of 2011, as I now call it. Paul and I were hosting our usual Passover Seder for our friends. For the uninitiated, Seder preparation is massive and I had been working a lot of hours at my job that week, so I decided to hire a helper from Task Rabbit to assist me in the kitchen.

Before the evening began, I showered, did my makeup and hair, looked at myself in the mirror and liked what I saw. Yup, I was lookin' good!

The doorbell rang and I greeted the Task Rabbit helper (let's call her "Sue") at the door. I introduced myself, showed her in and led her to the kitchen, where we began our work together.

Our ten guests began to arrive and I was particularly eager to meet Donna, the new girlfriend of our friend, Adam. She is a surgeon from Switzerland and sounded like a fascinating woman. I greeted Adam and Donna at the door. She was sweet and warm and we gave each other a hug even though we'd never met before. I went to hug Adam and instead of his usually warm greeting, he looked away, barely hugged me and quickly ran off to talk to someone else. Hmmm, strange. But I was too busy to worry about it in the moment. I had to go check on my matzo ball soup.

I went to the kitchen, chatted with Sue who was cutting the chicken and went to lift the lid on the simmering soup. I knew a cloud of steam would rise and instinctively, I leaned back so my prosthetic nose would not get a blast of heat. It was only then that I realized I had no nose on!

Oh my god! I had greeted all those people, including poor Sue who had no idea of my history, with the big honking hole in my face fully exposed to the world! Suddenly, Adam's reaction made sense. He was in the squeamish category. No wonder he didn't want to look at me!

In a loud voice, I yelled from the kitchen to Paul in the dining room in a way that everyone could hear, "Aitchy, why didn't you tell me I don't have a nose on?"

"Because you look normal to me!" he yelled back. It got a good laugh and I went immediately went and donned my very best nose, much to Adam's relief. Though somehow, every year on Passover, I manage to torment him with a reminder of that night.

The moral of the story: I thought I looked damn good when I checked my mirror before everyone arrived. Paul thought I looked perfectly fine. Clearly, the two of us have completely accepted me just as I am. How lucky am I to be able to say that?

*** *** ***

So, life goes on. I plan to be around for a long time – if COVID-19 doesn't get me – and the more years that pass, the less I care about not having a nose. For me, the aging process has brought a great freedom. I don't give a rat's ass what people think anymore.

Do I still miss my nose? Sure I do. If the opportunity arose to get one 3D-printed and attached, which is now being experimented with, I'd take it. But if that is never available in my lifetime – and it probably won't be – that's OK.

In the first chapter of this book, I talk about wondering why this happened to me and our conclusion that it was just the randomness of life. Sometimes shit just happens.

But it's what you do with the shit that's thrown at you that matters. I have not fundamentally changed who I am, and I knew I wouldn't. I have not become some great advocate for increasing melanoma awareness. I never did any public speaking or fundraising, or any of those things I would perhaps do if I were a more elevated version of myself. But I'm not. I'm just me.

The one thing I did do at the end of that first year was enter my information on a cancer site as a way of connecting with people who had gone through a similar experience. I was hoping to hear from others who might help me see my own future. But the opposite happened.

Over the years, I've heard from a handful of people about to lose their nose (or their loved ones) who were looking to me for the answers I had hoped to get myself all those years ago. And I've been happy to help with an email

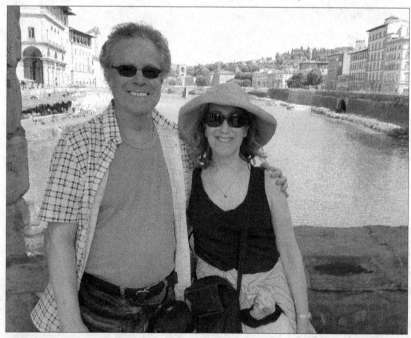

Happily Ever After

or a phone call. It seems to provide great relief to others to know I went through it and came out the other side to return to normal life.

Coincidentally, just this morning before sitting down to write this epilogue, I received an email from a woman in Nebraska whose husband is about to lose his nose. They were both – as one would expect – nervous about what was about to happen. We've now had a lovely exchange and I hope it helped her. I even sent her some pictures of me.

Maybe that's the best thing I can offer now as my way of giving back – information.

Reading back on my Caring Bridge entries now with hindsight, I can see how difficult it was to wake up each morning with so many unanswered questions and having no one to talk to who had been through the same experience.

So if I can make it easier for someone else it, I'm happy to do so – by answering an email, making a phone call or ...

... by writing this book!

ACKNOWLEDGEMENTS

There are a few special people who pushed me to do this book and helped me along through the process.

First, my never-ending gratitude to my oldest, dearest friend, Vicky Arenson Uhr. My best friend for over 60 years, she knows every great and rotten thing I've ever done in my entire life and still loves me. Thanks for reading my manuscript – multiple times – and offering your honest feedback to help me make it a better book.

Special thanks to Jami Seta Richards, Bob Melchionda and Seth Davis for their support and love and, well, you each know what you did!

Big thanks to my publisher and editor, Tom Brew. Thanks for enduring my obsession with ellipses and hyphenations. Your guidance and expertise were instrumental in always keeping me pointed in the right direction. You have my sincere gratitude.

Still and always to my dad, Herschel Caplan, once a journalist and always a lover of words, who I know would have been so happy I did this. My "thing for writing" was a genetic gift (or curse) directly from him.

And to all the underdogs and "dirty little freaks" out there who face the world each day missing body parts – we are "wrong in all the right ways," but to further quote Pink: We are all F***ing Perfect.

– Barbara

ABOUT THE AUTHOR

Barbara Caplan-Bennett has a degree in Literature from the University of Minnesota and a Certificate in Creative Writing from UCLA.

She has published essays and articles on a variety of subjects, as well as a novel, "Nothin' Left to Lose."

She lives in Chatsworth, California, with her husband, Paul, and they are owned by cats, William and Beckett, and Cally the Wonder Dog.

WHAT THEY'RE SAYING ABOUT 'NOSEWORTHY'

"Barbara Caplan-Bennett is also a brilliant writer who has written a personal, beautiful, compelling, wrenching and ultimately uplifting tale about things lost (her nose) and gained (badass optimistic attitude) – during her victorious fight over cancer. Treat yourself to the wisdom and eloquence contained in these pages. I promise you will love this book!"

– Seth Davis, CBS Sports college basketball analyst and author of several books, including "Wooden: A Coach's Life"

"Written with honesty, humor, and grace, Barbara Caplan-Bennett's "Noseworthy" takes us on a compelling journey with her from diagnosis to treatment to recovery. "Noseworthy" is a moving testament to resiliency of the human body and spirit."

– Lauren Maher, Licensed Marriage and Family Therapist

"Brave, honest, and funny. Barbara Caplan-Bennett found herself in a cage fight not only with cancer but with fear, vanity and self-worth. What she came out with is more than an inspirational survival story – it reads like the journal of a trusted friend."

– Cynthia Carle, co-writer THE SIXTH MAN, Humanitas Finalist YOU WISH

WHAT THEY'RE SAYING ABOUT 'NOSEWORTHY'

"Upon reading Ms. Caplan-Bennett's memoir, I am struck with one word: GRACE. If all of humankind could learn to handle their hardships with this degree of dignity, honesty and humor, the world would be a much better place. An inspiring must-read!"

— David Kaye, Owner, publisher and editor,
David Kaye Books & Memorabilia

"I really loved reading "Noseworthy." Barbara Caplan-Bennett is a talented writer, witty and endearing."

--Dana Escobar, LICSW

"Barbara Caplan-Bennett has the rare ability to make her readers feel like they are right there with her as she experiences every step of this unusual journey, from the initial shock and grief, through the ups and downs of the emotional recovery process, to ultimate acceptance.

"Through it all, she maintained her sense of humor, especially about some of the more absurd aspects of her situation. "Noseworthy" is a captivating book that is hard to put down and is a raw and honest depiction of psychological trauma, body image struggles, and the healing power of love."

-- Catherine Lamstein, Psy.D.

CPSIA information can be obtained
at www.ICGtesting.com
Printed in the USA
LVHW051647201120
672268LV00011B/1417